Award winning writer, television br[oadcaster and] activist, **Leslie Kenton** is well known [for her work in the] English-speaking world. Author of more than thirty best-selling books on health, personal development and spiritual power, her written works include *Journey to Freedom – 13 Quantum Leaps for the Soul, New Raw Energy, The Joy of Beauty, Passage to Power Journey to Freedom* and *Cook Energy*. She is described by the media as 'the guru of health and fitness': 'If there is one expert who can genuinely be described as pioneering and visionary, it's Leslie Kenton.'

Leslie's books have been translated into many foreign languages while her journalism has appeared in every national newspaper in Britain and many abroad. She was an Editor for *Harpers & Queen* magazine for fourteen years. Her network television series have included 'Raw Energy', a cookery series, and 'Ageless Ageing'. She has also written, made and presented a series of short films on health for the BBC. Recently Leslie turned her hand to photography, specializing in macro photographs. She has just completed her third fully illustrated photographic book.

Leslie lectures and teaches throughout the world, continually striving to bring to light natural methods of enhancing health, creativity and personal power to enable people to gain more control over their own lives and make better use of their personal creativity. Her **Journey to Freedom** workshops are now taught both in Europe and the Southern Hemisphere. She has always insisted that real health, creativity and personal power all come from within and that the only true 'guru' is the individual human soul. Leslie simply provides the tools that help people realise their own potential – improving their lives and having more to give to their families, communities and the planet itself.

Leslie has been a consultant to the European Parliament and a course developer for Britain's Open University. She has conceived and developed major cosmetic ranges and natural health care products for corporations throughout the world. Her work was honoured by her being asked to deliver the McCarrison Lecture at the Royal Society of Medicine and she has also received a number of awards for her work including the PPA 'Technical Writer of the Year'. Recently, her work has been increasingly concerned not only with the process of enhancing individual health but of helping to re-establish deep bonds of connectedness with the earth as a part of healing the planet. Leslie is the daughter of American Jazz musician, the late Stan Kenton.

Also by Leslie Kenton

LESLIE KENTON'S HEALING HERBS
TEN STEPS TO A NEW YOU
TEN STEPS TO A YOUNGER YOU
THE BIOGENIC FOOD COMBINING DIET
THE NEW ULTRAHEALTH
THE NEW JOY OF BEAUTY
TEN STEPS TO A NATURAL MENOPAUSE
PASSAGE TO POWER
THE NEW RAW ENERGY
RAW ENERGY RECIPES
CELLULITE REVOLUTION
THE NEW AGELESS AGEING
ENDLESS ENERGY
NATURE'S CHILD
LEAN REVOLUTION
JUICE HIGH
REJUVENATE NOW

QUICK FIX SERIES
Chill Out
Juice Blitz
Detox Now
Kick Colds

Fiction
LUDWIG (a spiritual thriller)

THE RAW ENERGY BIBLE

*Packed with raw energy goodness
and food combining facts*

Leslie Kenton

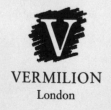

VERMILION
London

1 3 5 7 9 10 8 6 4 2

Original text copyright Raw Energy Food Combining Diet
© Leslie Kenton 1996
Original text copyright Juice High © Leslie Kenton and
Russell Kronin 1996
Original text copyright Raw Energy Recipes © Leslie and
Susannah Kenton 1998
Compilation copyright © Leslie Kenton 1998

This compilation first published in 1998 by Vermilion,
This edition published in 2001 by Vermilion,
an imprint of Ebury Press, Random House,
20 Vauxhall Bridge Road, London SW1V 2SA
www.randomhouse.co.uk

Random House Australia (Pty) Limited
20 Alfred Street, Milsons Point, Sydney,
New South Wales 2061, Australia

Random House New Zealand Limited
18 Poland Road, Glenfield, Auckland 10, New Zealand

Random House South Africa (Pty) Limited
Endulini, 5a Jubilee Road, Parktown 2193, South Africa

The Random House Group Limited Reg. No. 954009

Papers used by Vermilion are natural, recyclable products made from
wood grown in sustainable forests.

Printed and bound in Great Britain by
Cox and Wyman, Reading, Berks

A CIP catalogue record for this book is available from the British Library.

ISBN 0 09 185664 7

The Raw Energy Bible
Contents

Measurements & Quantities

I have given approximate measurements in the recipes as cupfuls (an ordinary cup holds about 225 ml or 8 fl. oz), tablespoons, teaspoons, pinches and so on. Each time you make a recipe it will be slightly different, which is the whole fun of cooking and eating. Where measuring is important, I have given the imperial measurement as well as the metric. Most of the recipes are designed to feed four people. As the quantities are approximate, the amounts can easily be adjusted to suit your own particular needs.

In the text I have mainly used metric measurements except where the original research was done in pounds and ounces, or the statistics were quoted in gallons or feet and inches. It would be artificial in those cases to convert to metric for the sake of it. Here are a few metric/imperial equivalents which you may find useful.

Weight			Length		
28 g	=	1 oz	2.5 cm	=	1 in
125 g	=	4 oz (¼ lb)	30 cm	=	1 ft
450 g	=	1 lb	1 m/100 cm	=	39 in/3.3 ft
1 kg	=	2.2 lb	1.6 km	=	1 mile

Volume		
600 ml	=	1 pint
1 litre	=	1¾ pints
4.5 litres	=	1 gallon

Author's Note

The material in is book is intended for information purposes only. None of the suggestions or information is meant in any way to be prescriptive. Any attempt to treat a medical condition should always come under the direction of a competent physician – and neither we nor the publisher can accept responsibility for injuries or illness arising out of a failure by a reader to take medical advice. We are only reporters. We also have a profound interest in helping ourselves and others to maximize potentials for positive health which include being able to live at a high level of energy, intelligence and creativity. For all three are expressions of harmony within a living, organic system.

Leslie Kenton
1998

Introduction

Raw foods have real power. The Raw Energy diet – in which between half and three-quarters of your food is eaten raw – enhances vitality, improves athletic performance, and regenerates the body in medically measurable ways. And by cleaning up your body and helping to restore metabolic balance, Raw Energy sets you on the path to better mental as well as physical health. The Raw Energy diet helps regenerate every organ and system thereby promoting feelings of well-being and recreating superb biochemical functions. This in turn helps to clear the mind and alleviate emotional distress.

A high raw or all raw diet is often used in healing by practitioners of natural medicine. They recognise that Raw Energy's health-enhancing power comes in part from the remarkable ability that raw foods have to encourage the elimination of wastes. Indeed, a raw food diet similar to the one described in this book forms the basis of detoxifying regimes in expensive spas throughout the world.

A high raw diet also provides optimal nutritional support for healing and high level health. When we cook and process our foods, many vital elements for health – including vitamins, minerals and proteins – are denatured or destroyed. A high raw diet, on the other hand, ensures that you get optimal levels of vitamins and minerals, fibre, easily assimilated proteins and top quality essential fatty acids.

So far, so good. The fact that detoxifying the body brings rejuvenation and that a fresh, crunchy carrot is frankly better for you than one whose natural goodness has been boiled away may come as no surprise to most people. These things are only part of the story.

Raw foods, it now appears, also contain a virtually unlimited variety of health-enhancing factors in pristine conditions. These range from *carotenoids* (which enhance the immune functions) and the powerfully detoxifying if unpronounceable *isothiocyannates* to *flavones* and *pycnogenols* (which inhibit the spread of cancer and guard against premature ageing). As nutritionists and biochemists identify more and more health-promoting plant compounds, the list of these factors – whose existence was undreamed of only a few years ago – grows longer by the week. The significant things to understand about these newly discovered plant factors is that they exist in perfect form, as Nature created them, in *raw* plants, not in cooked ones. The anti-ageing protective anti-oxidant properties of these plant factors is even greater than that of the now well-known anti-oxidant vitamins and minerals such as A, C, E and selenium.

Fresh, raw foods – vegetables and fruits, sprouted seeds and grains – also carry within them a phenomenal power that biophysicists call *energetic information*. The energetic properties of raw foods appear to play a vital role in enhancing the total health of the human body. Specifically, raw foods carry what the Swiss physician Max Bircher-Benner described as *quantum sunlight*. He explained this as a high level of 'order' from the sun's energy, which is converted by plants through photo-synthesis and stored in fresh, live foods. When we eat these foods we are able, literally, to 'drink order' – which means we can maintain a high level of energy and harmony in our bodies, and thereby resist the degenerative and entropic processes that affect all life on earth.

We still do not fully understand how the energetic

order that is present in a high raw diet actually works. Yet thousands of people around the world who have already incorporated raw food into their lives attest to its power. They know from experience that the Raw Energy way of eating does more for vitality, strength and good looks than any other single thing they can use to improve their health.

There is a widespread perception that good health is hard work. Well, you must actually *want* the payoff – better health than you ever thought you could achieve – to the point where you take the trouble to find and use the very best raw foods. But following a Raw Energy diet does not require stressful self-denial. Raw Energy recipes are mouth-watering. You won't go hungry: in fact you are likely to enjoy the sensual pleasures of good food even more than you do already. And you won't have to spend hours in the kitchen. Preparing Raw Energy foods and juices is simple, fun and a real aesthetic treat.

As we approach the millennium, we stand on the threshold of a revolution in nutrition – a revolution based on plant power. Raw Energy, which is all about fresh, organically grown, raw plants, sits right at the heart of the plant power revolution.

Recent research on the properties of plant foods and their dramatic effects on living organisms is ushering in a whole new era for natural health and healing. It will be exciting to see what further research reveals in the next decade or two. In the meantime the benefits of Raw Energy eating continue to dazzle those who experience them. By joining the Raw Energy movement, you are harnessing the power of Nature in a way that will help rejuvenate your body, revitalize your spirit and quite literally transform your life.

BOOK ONE:
RAW ENERGY FOOD COMBINING DIET

For Jean Morgan

who knows first hand the
blessings of food combining

Contents

THE PRINCIPLES

1
Simply the Best

Food combining really works. It is capable of taking excess weight off a body so simply it can be hard to believe. It can also help heal any number of long-standing ailments, from arthritis to depression, chronic fatigue, skin disorders and stomach ulcers. So good are the effects of food combining that it is little wonder the 'uninitiated' – including doctors and scientists who have never tried it – often find its beneficial results hard to swallow. How can something so simple do so much for so many? Food combining is also fun. Add the raw energy element to it and you create an unbeatable combination to help you tap into energy you never knew you had.

A little miracle of nature, the Raw Energy Food Combining Diet is the easiest and most pleasant way imaginable to shed excess fat without ever going hungry. In the process it can rejuvenate and regenerate a body and heighten vitality, making you look and feel great.

Perfect Past

Far from being some new fad, food combining diets have been tried and tested for almost two hundred years. In the last century they were used as a way of healing illness and of helping the body establish a high level of well-being. The American doctor William Howard Hay became famous for his food combining 'cures' – cures which he consistently attributed not to his own skills but to the skills of Nature herself. Once one learns to live within Her laws, he insisted, Her gifts to us are endless. Food combining was also widely taught by the Natural Hygienists in the United States and by that branch of the medical community in Europe working within the long tradition of nature-cure.

In recent times, public awareness of the importance of food combining has grown thanks to simple guide books, such as *Food Combining For Health* by Doris Grant and Jean Joice, and the American, Dr Herbert Sheldon's *Food Combining Made Easy*. Although there are often minor variations between them, each tradition which incorporates food combining as a tool for establishing radiant health or for fat loss uses the same core principles.

Aim for the Top

When it comes to weight-loss, the Raw Energy Food Combining Diet is the most effective diet of all. It adds the amazing properties of living foods to the simple technique of separating concentrated protein foods – such as eggs and cheese, meat and fish – at a meal, from concentrated carbohydrate foods – such as bread, cereals and potatoes. It is a system of living based on natural fresh foods – vegetables and fruits, wholegrains, seeds, nuts and eggs, with or without dairy products, fish, poultry and game.

Raw energy, where 50 per cent or more of your foods are eaten raw, has been used far longer than food combining – in fact for thousands of years – as a way of improving physical health and enhancing awareness throughout the civilized world. Raw Energy principles also form the basis of health and rejuvenation treatment at Europe's and America's finest health farms and spas. There, people pay a small fortune to have their bodies renewed. You can experience the same benefits of exclusive spas and health farms by using the Raw Energy Food Combining Diet at home and instead of having to pay through the nose for it, it can cost you only pennies.

Those who benefit from these spa treatments include women with cellulite, people whose metabolism has been drastically slowed down by indiscriminate use of nutritionally inadequate crash diets, and those who can't seem to shed fat at all except on starvation fare. They also include men and women who have difficulty shedding excess pounds because of food sensitivities and addictions and people who are riddled with guilt at what they see as their 'lack of self control'. By this I mean those of us who sit down to have one biscuit with a cup of tea only to find to our horror that we have devoured the whole packet. Finally, they include a few of us who, even on a healthy diet of natural foods, still have a tendency to hold on to the fat deposits in our bodies.

Go For Joy

The Raw Energy Food Combining Diet is as different from standard weight-loss regimes as a wild horse is from a taxi cab. There is nothing mechanical about it. Nor do you have to count calories or go hungry; unlike most diets, raw energy will never leave you looking haggard or feeling washed out. Instead it supports health and good looks in the highest possible way.

In fact, 'Raw energy' is an apt name for a way of eating and living which can enhance cellular vitality, restore healthy metabolism, put virtually endless energy at your disposal, and encourage your body to rebalance its biophysical and biochemical functioning so that it slowly but surely returns to its natural size and shape.

Real health cannot be measured by the absence of disease alone. It goes far beyond. Real health is not so much a *state* as a living *process* – a process through which you can make greater and greater use of your innate potential for creativity, aliveness and joy. Helping you get there is what the Raw Energy Food Combining Diet is all about.

Have you ever seen a young horse racing from one end of his field to another for the sheer pleasure of the feeling of movement in his body? Watching him move with dilated nostrils and mane blowing free can give you a real sense of what a high level of well-being – health in its broadest sense – is like: ease, freedom and above all *aliveness*.

Feel the Power

The Raw Energy Food Combining Diet can help you experience this. It has already helped thousands who have used it either because they needed to shed excess fat from their bodies or because they were less healthy than they wanted to be.

Michelangelo claimed that he never imposed any shape or form on to the piece of marble he was carving. He insisted that instead he simply used his sculptor's tools to *reveal the natural form hidden within* the stone. In many ways an overweight body is rather like his marble. Within it is hidden its vital, naturally healthy and lean form. Raw Energy Food Combining is nothing more than an efficient tool for helping to uncover it – a biological method of 'living sculpture'.

The idea that steady and permanent fat-loss can take place as a result of eating natural delicious foods while avoiding certain food combinations is going to come as a shock to some people – both nutritionists and laymen alike – who have been brought up to believe that counting calories and going hungry is the *only* way to shed excess weight. Old assumptions about weight-loss die hard. And, as you might imagine, such a diet is decidedly

unpopular with the multi-million pound slimming industry, which survives on people's failures – failures which
keep selling diet products almost as fast as they can be
manufactured. But it can be a godsend to people who
have struggled long with the battle of the bulge and who
genuinely want to get rid of fat which does not rightly
belong to them, and to 'run free' as the horse does.

A Whole New Ball Game

Grasp the basics of raw energy and you need never spend
hours poring over long lists of what goes with what or
fretting over whether or not the salad dressing contains
apple juice which may or may not go with your poached
fish. The diet is easy to put into practice. It is a question
of feeling your way into a new way of thinking about
meals. Once you familiarize yourself with which foods
belong in what general categories you will find it is child's
play to plan meals.

In this little book you will find all you need – recipes,
guidelines for a raw energy lifestyle, plus a fortnight of
meals to inspire you. There is also a reference list of
foods and categories and a chart to tell you what goes
best with what. Meanwhile, here are the first principles:

- Do not eat a concentrated starch food with a concentrated protein food at the same meal.
- Try to serve only one concentrated protein food or one
  concentrated starch food per meal.
- Leave at least four to five hours between a starch meal
  and a protein one and vice-versa.

First, let's look at the rhymes and reason most weight-
loss diets fail, then we'll get on to the good stuff – how to
make it all work.

2
The Body Strikes Back

Everybody who's ever read a diet book knows that slimming is supposed to be a piece of cake. The 'weight-loss gurus' tell us: 'One pound of fat is equal to 3,500 calories. Just tighten your belt, count your calories and subtract them from the number your body needs for energy.' (At this point they refer you to one of those dreary weight/height charts.) 'For each 3,500 calories you cut out you'll get a pound lighter. What could be easier?'

It Doesn't Work

It looks great on paper. Trouble is for most of us it just doesn't work. Why? Because nobody ever got fat just because they had a big appetite. Neither are you likely to achieve *permanent* slimness by counting calories alone.

The common myths about slimming are based on three beliefs. The first is the notion that weight-loss depends on the conscious mind balancing the body's energy intake and expenditure. The second is the idea that your body exerts no biological control over how much fat it stores. The third is the presumption that calorie-consumption is the significant factor in body-weight. All three beliefs support a multi-million pound slimming industry with all its hype, but all three are false – as dozens of scientific studies have shown.

The Slow Burn

What really determines weight-loss and maintaining it afterwards is not some abstract formula of calorie deprivation but rather how fast your body metabolizes – burns up – both the excess fat it is carrying and the food you take in day to day. This in turn largely depends upon how much cellular energy is available for the job and how efficient is your metabolism.

Sad to tell, the fatter you get, the slower your metabolic rate becomes – especially on a typical low-calorie slimming regime. In fact so inefficient can the metabolism of overweight people become that some who weigh more than 260 pounds can maintain their weight on as little as 1,000 calories a day.

The very act of going on a low-calorie diet slows your metabolism even further: your body learns to conserve energy because it feels thrown into a situation of potential starvation. This leads to rebound eating as natural hunger breaks through the constraints of personal resolve. Research carried out since the turn of the century has confirmed all of this over and over again. Yet it is something diet books still conveniently choose to ignore.

Lay the Guilt

Instead they tend to push some kind of guilt trip on people. They make you feel that you are lacking will-power or perseverance if, after ten days on some 1,000-calorie regime, you feel sluggish, slow, tired and dull, and then break your diet in a desperate attempt to restore energy and regain a sense of comfort.

Diet books are also very deceptive about the initial rapid weight-loss which most experience during the first few days on a regime. They encourage you to believe that this is good evidence that the crash diet you are on is working and that it will continue to work so long as you have the 'will-power' to keep at it. The truth is that what has been lost from your body in the first few days is not fat but water. Once this excess water from your tissues has been shed, weight-loss slows dramatically. It may even stop altogether because your metabolism has been slowed by the diet so you are simply not burning fat.

Yet it is *fat* you want to shed, not just water and certainly not lean muscle tissue. Otherwise your body will get flabbier and flabbier while your metabolism – not to mention your overall vitality – will become further depressed. There are hundreds of thousands of people who lose the same five or ten pounds over and over again only to gain it all back within a few weeks or months.

Go For Order

To shed fat *forever* you must re-establish biological and energetic *order* in your body. For it is a disturbance in this order that has caused it to accumulate in the first place. As this happens, not only does your metabolism function normally again, your digestion improves, chronic fatigue becomes a thing of the past and all those cravings that once led you to eat the wrong foods or more food than your body needs, vanish. Sounds too good to be true? Then you have not yet experienced the powers of nature-cure.

Nature-cure is an ancient system of healing which uses simple things like food and water, sleep and exercise, to establish the highest possible level of biological and energetic order in any organism. This allows an ailing or distorted body to heal itself, restoring to its owner a high level of energy, health and good looks – naturally.

The weight-loss which occurs on the Raw Energy Food Combining Diet is nothing more than simple nature-cure. It is one of the signs that your body is restoring itself to its more normal shape and function. And the power of such a diet by no means ends at paring away excess fat from an overweight body. It has also been shown to encourage the healing of any number of minor and major illnesses from rheumatoid arthritis to cancer. As any expert in natural medicine will tell you, it sets up the best possible conditions for all of this to happen. A major part of bringing all of these wonderful things about is the diet's ability to detoxify the body, while a major reason that both overweight and illness become seeded in any body is the build-up of toxicity in the system.

Toxic Traumas

The standard and widely held view of fat stored in the body is that it is fundamentally 'passive'. It just sort of sits there happily conserving energy and insulating you against cold and shock. The fact is, our fat-stores have a very *active* role to play – a protective role which it is vital to understand if you are to shed fat permanently. Fat-stores gather substances which the body experiences as toxic or poisonous and tuck them out of harm's way.

Fat cells are the perfect storehouse for these wastes since they are much less metabolically active than other cells in your body. (This is also why, once fat has been stored in cells, it can be very difficult to budge.) People who easily store fat often have difficulty dealing with these wastes. Gradually a vicious circle is created: fat-stores lower metabolic rate. Toxins continue to build up. The liver, whose job it is to cleanse them, is put under stress. This makes it increasingly difficult to eliminate them and even more difficult for you to avoid laying down yet more fat.

Ask Any Rat

A major reason why there is so much obesity in our society is that we eat so many junk foods. Feed the same foods to rats and 60 to 70 per cent of them get fat. It has nothing to do with will-power, sin or guilt. Junk foods – indeed, all refined convenience foods – are not only nutritionally unable to support a high level of health, they contain lots of sugar and white flour, chemical colourings, preservatives and flavourings, all of which encourage the build-up of wastes in the body in quantities greater than your normal waste-elimination channels can handle.

When we eat convenience foods over a period of time two things happen. First, we end up with subclinical nutritional deficiencies of vitamins and minerals because so many essential nutrients have been lost in the processing and storage of these foods. Second, wastes accumulate in the tissues. Those of us who have inherited a genetic tendency to lay down fat-stores grow fatter. Meanwhile, the subclinical deficiencies that we have slowly developed in consuming typical western fare tend to create chronic fatigue, contribute to poor skin tone and the laying down of cellulite in women. It also predisposes us to early ageing and further slows metabolism.

Accumulated wastes are stored mostly in the body's fat cells. The more wastes you have the bigger your fat cells get and the fatter you can become, whatever valiant efforts you may make to change things. It is little wonder that excess fat deposits have become such a problem as we approach the millennium if you consider the toxicity to which we are exposed. Industrial wastes fill our rivers and seas, and quite literally billions of gallons of chemicals are poured on our crops and farmlands every year. Even the fat of Arctic seals has been shown to be permeated by chemical poisons such as DDT.

Energy Equations

There is one more thing which you should know about a body which has a high level of wastes stored in its cells. Much of the available energy in such a system tends to be channelled into trying to handle these toxins instead of into keeping cells functioning at a high level of competence and efficiency as in a truly healthy lean body. In broad terms this means that you are likely to experience flagging vitality over the years and to feel that you simply can't make the effort to change things for the better.

To achieve permanent fat-loss you need rational and effective methods for eliminating toxic wastes from your body, for enhancing metabolic functions and for eliminating cravings. Once you have accomplished these goals you need to follow a way of living afterwards which will permanently help prevent their build-up. The Raw Energy Diet combines well-proven techniques of food combining with a high-raw way of eating, rich in living foods, to do all three. It boosts your metabolism and detoxifies your body while protecting your system from the build-up of acid wastes in the blood which can trigger binge eating. It alkalinizes the system and helps restore metabolic balance. It also helps resolve the energy crises which takes place when a body is overweight and digestion is overtaxed. Best of all, once the detox experience is well under way, it can bring you to experience a whole new kind of energy that will have you looking good and feeling great day after day.

3
Energy Crisis

Your body expends more energy on the digestion of food than on any other function. This is one of the main reasons why after a big meal you can feel sluggish or sleepy and experience a lowering of vitality. What has happened is that your body has had to redirect blood (and therefore energy) away from the brain and other organs towards the gut, where your basic life-force is now busy breaking down the food you have eaten and transforming it into chemicals which can be absorbed into your bloodstream for use by your cells. In fact, the amount of energy needed to digest food is even greater than that which you use when taking strenuous exercise.

Energy Equations

For the slimmer serious about shedding fat permanently, the question of how his or her energy is directed becomes a very important issue. For an abundance of steadily available energy is needed to carry out the vital task of detoxification on which fat-loss depends. This is why all the foods you eat should be digested as efficiently as possible, both to preserve your vitality and also to make sure the quantity of toxic wastes created as byproducts during the process is minimal.

The standard western meal consisting of meat-and-two-veg plus bread, potatoes and a dessert represents just about the worst way you can eat if you want to lose weight. This has nothing to do with how high in calories it is either. The slimmers' low-calorie version is little better. It is the kind of meal which presents your digestive system with the most difficult of all foods for it to break down and make use of: a concentrated protein, here in the form of meat, taken together with a concentrated starch in the form of bread and potatoes.

Spanner in the Works

The human body is simply not designed to digest efficiently more than one concentrated food in the stomach at the same time. An awareness of this principle lies at the basis of virtually every tradition of natural healing.

What is meant by 'concentrated'? Any food which does *not* come into the category of a 'high-water food'. (More about the importance of the high-waters in a little while.) In other words we are talking about any food which is neither a fresh raw vegetable nor a fresh raw fruit.

Less Than Perfect

The usual response to this information goes something like this: 'How ridiculous! I have been eating meat-and-two-veg for 40 years and done perfectly well on it.' Perhaps. Yet just how well is 'perfectly well'?

If forced to be completely honest, most people who have been living in such a way for 25 to 40 years or longer will tell you they experience any number of minor digestive problems, from indigestion and flatulence to persistent hunger and being overweight, not to mention more serious rheumatoid conditions and other chronic ailments that can develop over decades of subjecting the digestive system to the heavy strain of having to cope with concentrated starches and proteins at the same meal.

The Four Horsemen

Our so-called 'normal' way of eating in the west has four basic problems when it comes to fat shedding. First, it puts great strain on your body's enzyme system – the system responsible for food breakdown and assimilation. It simply does not respect your body's enzyme limitations – and everyone's are different, depending on their genetic inheritance and on how nutritionally adequate a diet you were raised on (more about enzymes in a moment). Second, it makes heavy demands on available energy and vitality – energy which is very much needed to carry out the detoxification processes needed for permanent fat-loss. Third, it tends to produce excessive quantities of biochemical wastes which further add to the toxicity you must clear from your system if you are to be permanently free of excess fat-stores. Finally, the average diet does not supply a full complement of vitamins, minerals, trace elements, and essential fatty acids needed to support health.

So, while the human organism has a remarkable ability to adapt to difficult circumstances, and you may indeed live reasonably well on meals of concentrated starch with concentrated protein for many years, you have probably not lived this way without paying a price for it, even if the price paid so far is only decreased vitality and having to carry about with you more fat than you would like to have.

Break Down

All of the changes to foods which take place during digestion – the processes by which foods are broken down into their constituent chemical parts for use by the cells – take place thanks to enzymes. An enzyme is a kind of physiological catalyst which depends upon the presence of certain vitamins and minerals to do its job of making things happen biochemically. Each enzyme in your body is quite specific in its action. The enzymes which act upon starches do not and cannot affect either proteins or fats.

Different classes of enzymes, such as those which help break down starchy foods and those which help to break down proteins, need different chemical environments too. Starch-digesting enzymes need an alkaline environment. Protein-digesting enzymes need an acid medium: they cannot function in an alkaline environment. This is why eating high-protein foods such as eggs or meat stimulate the body's production of hydrochloric acid which, in turn, acts on the substance pepsinogen, secreted by the gastric glands, to produce the enzyme pepsin for splitting proteins. But the process only takes place efficiently in an acid environment. If there are any concentrated starches or sugars present in a meal, the accompanying alkalinity, passed on as they began to be broken down by saliva in the mouth, interferes with the process.

This can and often does result in proteins being incompletely and inefficiently digested. If the situation is severe enough it can result in 'food allergies', aches and pains and even emotional abberations – all the consequence of incompletely digested proteins (which even in minute quantities are toxic to the blood) being drawn in through the wall of the gut. On the other hand, enzymes needed to break down the starches of bread require just the opposite environment – a mildly alkaline medium. In fact they can often be destroyed even in a mildly acid milieu.

Starchy Truths

Starch digestion begins in the mouth, through the action of the starch-splitting enzyme ptyalin which prepares the starches for their journey into the small intestine, where their main digestion takes place. The role of ptyalin in starch digestion is extremely important: all starchy foods need to be chewed thoroughly so that saliva (which is mildly alkaline) and the ptyalin it contains can break them down sufficiently for the small intestine to carry on the good work after they are swallowed. If this doesn't happen then similar food sensitivities can occur.

The good news is that when people with food sensitivities learn the art of food combining, and practise it, many worrying and oppressive symptoms lift away. Separating concentrated protein foods and concentrated starches – that is taking them at different meals – you take the pressure off digestion, reduce the build-up of toxicity and free energy.

There is no great magic to it. By making such a change you begin to eat in a way that shows respect for the body's enzymic limitations. You are helping your body to digest your foods fully and properly – sometimes for the first time in one's life. And complete and efficient digestion is absolutely essential if you are permanently to rid yourself of the burden of unwanted fat forever. Meanwhile, plenty of fresh raw foods each day makes the job even easier.

Live for the Liver

The liver is your body's chemical factory. It carries out a myriad of essential functions, from storing vitamins and metabolizing fats to destroying unwanted materials and providing enzymes for many of your body's chemical processes. One of the most important of these functions is the breaking down or metabolism of toxic wastes. Living foods help your liver to do this job. The liver has a quite phenomenal capacity to handle detoxification. But, when it is living under constant strain as a result of having to recycle more wastes than it can manage, as well as trying to carry out all of its other functions at the same time, it can become 'overloaded' so that it simply is no longer equal to the task. Then toxins – the majority of which are fat-soluble – are simply shunted via the blood and lymph to be stored in your cells as fat.

A liver which has become chronically overloaded as its owner continues to eat the wrong kind of foods and drink the wrong kind of drinks (or to eat and drink them in the wrong combinations) will progressively send more and more toxins towards the fat cells for safe storage.

Unlike most diets, the Raw Energy Food Combining Diet works *with* the liver. That's where fruit comes in. The liver is most active between midnight and midday, so the diet uses only fruits for breakfast. Fresh fruits are so easily digested that unlike cooked foods, concentrated starches and proteins, they don't require work from the liver to handle them. This leaves your liver free to get on with the job of deep cleansing your body and shedding fat. Hence the fruit rule:

Eat fruit on its own or leave at least 20 minutes between a fruit appetizer and the next course of your meal.

4
Life Power

Living foods have special properties for weight-loss. This is a truth which is nothing less than mind-blowing for most people. We have been brought up to consider food only in terms of chemical categories such as protein, carbohydrate, fats and fibre and to measure energy only in terms of calories.

Biochemical Blockbusters

Fresh fruits and vegetables, sprouted seeds and grains and pulses, offer the highest complement of vitamins and minerals, essential fatty acids, easily assimilated top-quality protein, fibre and wholesome carbohydrate found in nature. Such a natural complement of nutrients in superbly balanced form supplies your body with the substances it needs for its metabolic biochemical reactions to function at a high level of efficiency. This is exactly what you want to encourage – steady and permanent fat-loss.

In an overweight body, metabolism has often become sluggish and inefficient, eating the wrong foods or foods in poor combinations means vitality has been lowered and subclinical nutritional deficiencies have developed as a result of having lived on a less-than-optimal diet over a period of years.

A diet replete with living foods is the quickest and most effective way to restore balance and normality. The power that fresh, raw, living foods hold to transform life, health and good looks, lies outside the awareness of most classic nutritionists and biochemists busy quantifying the chemical characteristics of proteins, carbohydrates, and fats, with vitamins and minerals. Most of them also still tend to think in mechanistic ways.

However, the health-enhancing properties of living foods have long been tested and eulogized by highly respected European and American physicians – from Gordon Latto and Philip Kilsby in Britain, Max Bircher-Benner in Switzerland and Max Gerson in Germany, to Henry Lindlahr and J.H. Tilden in the United States.

Subtle Energies

Now, thanks to recent research into the electromagnetic and energetic properties of living plant cells, we are beginning to formulate a scientific explanation of *how* living foods can be so beneficial for enhancing health and encouraging natural weight-loss. We are beginning to understand that there is more to the metabolic improvements effected by living foods than can be measured through biochemical means alone.

All energy comes from the sun. It gets into our foods through the process of photosynthesis which plants carry out: they take in water and carbon dioxide and, thanks to enzymes they contain, in the presence of chlorophyll they produce carbohydrates (which we eat) and oxygen.

We get three types of energy from our food: kinetic energy for motion; electrical energy to maintain cell-wall integrity, muscle and nerve impulses; and chemical energy for the manufacture, storage and transport of chemicals for metabolic processes. Sunlight, through photosynthesis in plants, is the primary source of all three. This fact, although widely known and completely accepted, is too often forgotten when considering the kind of energetic information needed for high-level health which is brought to us through the foods we eat.

Sunlight Quanta

The great European physician Max Bircher-Benner, who was an expert on the healing properties of fresh live foods, always insisted that, because raw foods were still living, they contained a special health-enhancing quality of energy directly derived from the sun during photosynthesis. It is a kind of energy which is destroyed when foods are cooked or processed. When we eat these foods, he said, this special energy is passed on to us. He referred to it as 'sunlight quanta' or 'life-force'. By and large Bircher-Benner's assertions were pooh-poohed by the scientists of his day. Now physicists, many biochemists and a growing number of nutritionists, consider there is great truth in what he taught. For the biological 'information' for health and life which passes to us through the foods we eat is by no means of a *chemical* nature alone. Research into physics and the new biology demonstrates that there are other subtle forms of energy which animate organisms carried in living systems, plants and animals. These subtle energies play a central part in enhancing metabolism, rebalancing your body's functions and eliminating excess fat-stores.

Recently, thanks to the work of many highly respected biologists who have been looking both at just what kind of 'information' comes to us through the foods we eat and the subtle energies present in our environment, we have begun to measure such things as electrical fields in living cells. Evidence has emerged from this work to show that the electromagnetic or subtle energy properties of living food and of the body itself are central to how well metabolism functions and how healthy we are.

In the United States, Robert O. Becker, an orthopaedic surgeon, nominated for a Nobel Prize for his work on the regeneration of tissue using electromagnetic fields, has discovered that electric conduction mechanisms in the body appear to form the basis of control systems in living organisms, and that the metabolic functions of living cells can be significantly influenced by electromagnetic means. Other scientists such as F.S.C. Northrop and Harold Saxton Burr showed the presence of what they call 'life fields' or 'L-fields' around seeds. By measuring the intensity of L-fields they are able to predict how healthy or unhealthy plants grown from them will be. They have also found that, when seeds are subjected to chemicals or heated, their fields become significantly weaker – in Bircher-Benner's terms, losses in sunlight quanta or life-force have taken place.

Living Light

Very recently, a highly respected German scientist, Fritz-Albert Popp, in collaboration with a team in China has shown – just as Bircher-Benner taught – that living cells of plants emit light in the form of biophoton radiation and that in the process of dying, as when we eat them, their cells radiate this light very intensely. Meanwhile, American cancer researcher, Herbert A. Pohl, has shown that living cells produce natural alternating-current (AC) fields which reflect biological events necessary for cell metabolism, health and growth.

Doctors and scientists working with raw energy to restore health and normal weight to patients have long been aware that many of the reasons why living foods such as fresh raw fruits and vegetables, and life-generating foods such as seeds and sprouts are so beneficial for reducing fat deposits will only begin to be explained fully when we have a better grasp of exact mechanisms by which the subtle energies in living foods act upon our bodies to encourage detoxification, to heighten enzyme activity, to improve cellular metabolism, to encourage fat-burning and to foster the quite marvellous kind of internal living sculpture which can restore some of the most neglected of overweight bodies to their natural leaner form.

It may be years before we have a full understanding of what is going on, while someone on a raw energy diet begins to reap the rewards of a slimmer, firmer body and a healthier, more energetic way of being. In fact, we will probably never have the full answer, although the work of scientists such as Becker, Popp and Pohl is rapidly taking us nearer that goal.

In this way a raw energy way of eating encourages biochemical functions in your body to return to normal. It also fosters a high level of health and good looks. That is why, depending upon how rapidly you want to lose weight (and there are strong indications that you should not lose weight at a rate faster than two pounds a week if you intend to keep it off permanently), raw foods should form between 50 and 75 per cent of your food combining diet. Accomplishing this is easier (and more delicious) than you think.

New Steps

Week by week, scientists take giant steps forward in understanding how Raw Energy works its miracles. Plants, we are learning, seem to contain a virtually unlimited variety of health-enhancing substances and compounds. When vegetables and fruits are eaten raw, these compounds work in synergy to keep you radiant and well.

Here are just a few of the newly discovered plant factors that are present in great abundance in a Raw Energy diet:

- Pine bark and fresh vegetables and fruits, notably grape seeds, contain **pycnogenols**, which you may also find called catechins, procyanadins and epicatechins. As well as being powerful protectors against cancer and premature ageing, the pycnogenols strengthen capillaries and help rebuild collagen and connective tissue in the skin and the body as a whole. Scientists have established that pycnogenol is 20 times more effective in quenching harmful free radicals than vitamin C. Pycnogenol can even help protect skin cells from damage by ultraviolet radiation.

- **Flavonoids,** commonly called bioflavonoids, also inhibit cancer and early ageing. They are found in many fruits, such as grapefruits, oranges, apples and tangerines where they appear as rutin, quercetin and tangeretin. Many of the flavonoids also have anti-inflammatory effects, helping to lessen allergic responses by inhibiting the release of histamine. A recent report in *The Lancet* highlighted the results of a Dutch study which concluded that elderly men with a high intake of five flavonoids have a significantly reduced risk of dying from heart disease.

- Cruciferous vegetables such as cabbage, cauliflower, broccoli and Brussels sprouts are rich in **isothiocyannates,** which also have anti-ageing and anti-cancer properties. A further class of compounds, known as **indoles,** is also present in these vegetables. Indoles detoxify the body of petrochemically derived oestrogen mimics in the environment, enhance your ability to deal with stress and improve your immune functions.

- Richly coloured vegetables and fruits contain **carotenoids** such as luetin, zeaxanthin and cryptoxanthin together with the more widely known beta carotene. Carotenoids are highly active in living organisms. As well as enhancing the immune functions and protecting the skin from free radical damage, they help clear toxic wastes, prevent premature degeneration and have a beneficial effect on eyesight.

5
Water Margin

We are part of a living planet whose surface is over 70 per cent water. The tissues of the human body are also more than 70 per cent water. To help restore true biochemical balance and metabolic functioning to a body burdened with excess fat it is important to eat plenty of foods which are high in water content.

Living Water

Fresh uncooked fruits and vegetables and sprouted seeds, grains and legumes are high in a special kind of water – the water naturally found in living cells. The water found in living foods is invaluable in helping your body transport nutrients to all its cells and in removing toxic wastes from them. In fact, it is quite different from the water which pours from your tap. Water in living foods carries electrolytes, vitamins, organic minerals, proteins, enzymes, amino acids, carbohydrates, natural sugars, fatty acids, and other nutrients vital in the restoration of high-level functioning to the body. It helps heighten cell metabolism and makes fat burning possible.

On the Raw Energy Food Combining Diet, between 50 and 75 per cent of the foods you eat while shedding excess fat should be foods of high-water content rather than foods from which the water has been removed through drying, baking, cooking and processing.

Most of the foods we in the west eat are either not high-water foods or they have had their natural water denatured and drained away by cooking. This includes breads and pastas, meat and cheese, fried potatoes and snack foods. Even when chosen from whole natural foods and prepared without chemical additives, low-water foods should be limited while you are shedding fat. Only high-water-content foods such as fresh raw fruits and vegetables are good at waste elimination.

Limit Low-Water Foods

Low-water-content foods act differently on your body from their high-water cousins. When a food's natural water content is removed by cooking or processing, the food changes the way it acts upon the body. Low-water foods tend to clog waste elimination mechanisms and to make you feel heavy and lethargic. Low-water foods also increase cravings for more food and force you to muster the most phenomenal will-power to keep from eating too much. It is the kind of will-power that can be sustained only for limited periods, which is why so many people are off-again-on-again when it comes to weight-loss diets.

It is important to restrict the low-water-content foods you eat to no more than 20 to 25 per cent of your diet while your body is burning excess fat. Later, when you have shed your fat and your metabolism is working in top form, you can incorporate more low-water-content foods into your diet if you want to (provided, of course, you choose the most wholesome of those available).

Drink Your Fill

What about that old adage which suggests drinking eight glasses of water a day? It is good advice for weight loss. It quite specifically helps compensate for the water-loss which occurs in the preparation of concentrated, cooked and processed foods which most people eat most of the time. But when more than 50 per cent of your foods are high-water-content and eaten in their natural fresh state, you don't need to worry so much about consuming masses of water. Of course, water acts as a natural appetite suppressant so go ahead if you fancy it. It also helps cleanse your body so drink as much fresh spring water as you like – provided, of course, you are not suffering from a kidney disease or other medical condition which precludes it.

Foods For Stamina

The rest of the Raw Energy Food Combining Diet consists of wholegrains, cooked vegetables, legumes, cooked eggs, dairy products (if you must) or fresh fish, organic meat, poultry or game. Although these foods offer little in the way of heightening cell vitality or detoxifying the body for fat-loss, they are delicious and satisfying to the palate. They are also good wholesome sources of proteins, vitamins and minerals. They are the foods which athletes or people doing hard physical work will want to eat enough of – particularly the grains. They make a rich and delicious contrast to the lighter, finer taste and feel of living foods. They will form the rest of your diet while you are slimming. Once you have lost the fat you want to shed, you can increase your intake of the stamina foods to 50 per cent or even more if you like. Many who have experimented with raw energy principles, however, find that restricting the intake of heavier foods to about 30 to 40 per cent of their diet makes them feel and look better permanently.

Shun the Destroyers

Health-destroying foods are those which, if taken in quantity, undermine health, distort biochemical balance in the body and foster degeneration and illness. The list of foods with health-destroying tendencies is a long one and getting longer every day as scientists discover new ways in which the chemical additives in convenience and processed foods, and the hormones and drugs given to the animals from which much of our meats are taken, pose threats to human health. They include foods which have been fragmented and excessively altered from their natural state such as foods made from white flour, refined sugar, and highly processed oils and margarines – in short any food whose vital nutrients have been depleted or destroyed. Not only do you want to avoid these foods because they put a damper on the cellular life processes which are so important in heightening metabolism and burning stored fat, but also because they are the most polluting of all foods. Enough said about what to avoid. Now let's look at the upside. You will be amazed to learn what the magic living foods offer in the way of natural appetite control.

6
Hunger Busting

Probably the worst thing any slimmer ever has to face is the feeling of never being satisfied. Persistent hunger is a major reason why people on conventional slimming diets never seem able to shed excess fat permanently. So common is it, not only with overweight people but with many of their slim brothers and sisters as well, that it is important to understand why it occurs and what can be done to get rid of it. Excessive hunger can have many causes – both emotional and physiological. But by far the most common (and the most often ignored) is chronically disturbed digestion.

Junk Food Makes You Hungry

If you have been eating irregularly, eating more than your body needs, eating foods full of chemically altered fats or which are refined and over-processed, then your natural appetite becomes distorted. To what extent depends both on the kind of digestive system you've inherited and on how badly, in physiological terms, it has been abused. Virtually every overweight body is a nutritionally starved body despite the number of calories it has consumed over the years. Its endocrine system, circulation, bones and nerves remain under constant stress. So does its digestive system.

The digestive system of a person who has been living on highly processed, chemically altered foods, or someone who chronically overeats, cannot function normally because it remains in a state of persistent stimulation. It experiences the constant overproduction of digestive juices. Good digestion is impaired. The body does not receive an adequate supply of vitamins and minerals – called *co-factors* – needed to trigger enzyme reactions. Many people in this state experience chronic hunger as a physical expression of subclinical nutritional deficiencies. The cells of their bodies are, in effect, crying out for nourishment which is not being adequately supplied. The body, in an attempt to rectify matters, seems to want to eat more and more. Another consequence is a slow-down in metabolic machinery, for every step in the body's metabolic processes depends upon good enzymic functions.

Tummy Troubles

In the beginning chronic overeating or eating the wrong kind of foods results in an over-acidic or irritated stomach. In time, however, this turns into a slack, acid-poor stomach with the kind of chronic inflammation of the intestines and bile duct that tends to accompany such a state. It is a series of events which occurs in almost every case of chronic overweight. It is also typical of people who suffer from food sensitivities.

Food sensitivities frequently accompany being overweight. The woman who reaches for that biscuit to go with her cup of tea and finds herself eating the whole pack is experiencing the kind of allergy-addiction which forms the basis of food and chemical sensitivities. Such 'food allergies' contribute greatly to weight-gain, not only because they stimulate people to eat far too much – particularly of those foods to which they are sensitive, but also because eating foods to which you are sensitive produces a very high level of toxic wastes – far more than your liver and your lymphatic system can efficiently eliminate. So what happens? Your body lays down yet more fat-stores to lock these toxins out of harm's way.

Back to Normal

Vital factors in achieving permanent fat-loss are the restoration of your digestive processes to normal and the elimination of the kind of chronic digestive irritation which fosters persistent overeating as well as a myriad of other problems, including excessive toxicity and impaired microcirculation. The taking of oral contraceptives and a wide range of other substances, from marijuana to common prescriptive drugs, including tranquillizers, can also contribute to the toxicity, forcing fat deposits to collect on those of us with a genetic tendency towards them.

Banish the Binge

This is where binge eating comes in too – with all the guilt, disappointment and misery which accompany it. Binge eating is a typical response to the kind of biochemical anguish caused by your bloodstream having been flooded with more toxic wastes than it can deal with all at once. These same wastes in the bloodstream – most of which are acidic – are also responsible for the common dieter's nervousness, which can also trigger the eating of undesirable foods in an attempt to gain comfort or a sense of relaxation. When dieters get the typical hang-overs and headaches it is simply a sign that the toxic wastes which were stored in your fat cells have now temporarily returned to the bloodstream to haunt you until they are eliminated from the body.

Bye-Bye Biscuits

Raw Energy Food Combining is the ideal antidote. First it gradually eliminates cravings by supplying your body with all the nutrients it needs (at least 50 essential nutrients are so far known. Living foods probably contain many more). Also, a diet high in raw foods calms an irritated and overactive digestive system so that its functions can gradually return to normal and you eliminate the ravenous hunger.

The result of all this is that the raw energy way of eating brings with it its own brand of natural appetite control. On a diet high in living foods the improvements which take place in digestion as well as the loss of weight itself occur steadily – quite naturally – without your having to pay attention to calories. Another wonderful thing about shedding excess fat this way is that you do not end up looking drawn or flabby. Skin and muscles become firmer and the whole body undergoes a slow process of regeneration which can seem quite miraculous to someone experiencing it.

Power For Order

Experts in the use of a high raw diet insist that the enzymes in raw fruits and vegetables also improve digestion since they *support* the body's own enzyme systems. Each food contains just the enzymes and co-factors (vitamins or minerals linked to an enzyme) needed to break down that particular food. When we destroy these enzymes by cooking or processing our foods, then our body has to make more of its own digestive enzymes in order properly to digest and assimilate them. Unless you have inherited a super-virile enzyme-replication system, without the enzymes from raw foods your body's own enzyme-producing abilities tend to wane, so that you make fewer and fewer enzymes as the years pass. Making sure your body has plenty of enzymes from raw foods is another way to help protect yourself from the food sensitivities and chronic digestive disturbances which lead to overeating.

Holistic Help

The whole issue of how digestion affects the build-up of fat-stores in the body and how it can help mobilize them is a complex one. One of the reasons why the Raw Energy Food Combining Diet is so effective is that, like any other natural form of treatment, it does not act on the body only in one or two specific ways. A diet high in living foods affects your body all over – *holistically* – in so many positive ways which interact and reinforce each other that it is impossible to delineate them all. It would even be pointless to try. The important thing is to experience for yourself just what all of these rather technical things mean in very simple terms: more energy, and freedom from constant hunger and from fatigue. It is fun to watch your body undergo its own process of living sculpture – reshaping itself from within as only a truly vital and healthy body can. Enjoy it.

7
A Question of Diet

To most people, embarking on the Raw Energy Food Combining Diet is a whole new experience. They often have questions. Here are the ones most frequently asked.

Q: You say it is not necessary on the Raw Energy Food Combining Diet to eat flesh foods. But without meat, how will I be sure that I am getting enough protein?

A: It is a common misconception that if you don't eat meat, poultry, fish, seafood and game, or plenty of dairy products, such as milk, cheese and eggs, then you won't get enough protein. This is simply untrue. Meat, like eggs and cheese, is often called a 'complete' protein. What this means is that it contains all the essential amino acids – those which your body cannot make itself – in a good balance so that once its protein is broken down into its constituent amino acids it will provide your system with the raw materials needed to build its own proteins. That is, to make new enzymes and hormones and to build muscle tissue. For many years nutritionists believed that we needed to take in all of the essential amino acids at each meal in order to make proper use of them – hence the idea that a 'complete protein' was essential. Now we know that this is simply not so. You can either take in all of the essential amino acids at one meal or you can take in some essential amino acids, say, from a grain food at one meal and others from vegetables at another meal and you will still get the equivalent of a complete protein food. In other words, your body will still be able with ease to make use of the aminos these food contain to build its own proteins.

You will notice that the Raw Energy Diet is not *high* in protein but *moderate* in protein. This is for a very good reason: a prolonged intake of too much protein tends to result in deficiencies of many essential minerals such as calcium, iron, zinc and phosphorous, and even some vitamins. Also many animal studies have now shown conclusively that, while a high-protein diet brings about early rapid growth, it can also result in early and rapid ageing and degeneration. Moderate protein intake is best for long term health and resistance to early ageing.

Q: How fast will I lose weight on the Raw Energy Diet?

A: That depends on the idiosyncrasies of your metabolism and on how rapidly your body detoxifies itself. In the beginning you will probably lose weight very quickly. But this initial weight-loss will be not fat but water as your system begins to clear of toxicity. (Wastes in the tissues encourage the body to retain water in order to dilute them and render them less dangerous.) It is best to aim for no more than two pounds lost a week. This way you give your body time to change gradually: you neither risk your system being flooded with toxicity (which can make you want to eat foods in combinations you should avoid) and nor do you trigger the 'setpoint' mechanisms that spur the body to regain weight lost.

In practice you may not have much choice in the matter since many people following a raw energy lifestyle lose weight *much* faster. If you find yourself shedding weight simply increase the foods you are eating cooked – a helpful way to slow down weight loss.

Q: The diet contains a lot of raw foods and I understand that raw foods are more difficult to digest. Will they give me problems such as flatulence or loose bowels?

A: This is a common misconception. Provided they are well chewed, raw foods are *less* difficult to digest than their counterparts: this is why they form the basis of traditional dietary treatments in natural medicine. Remember, all the uncooked foods you will be eating are rich in enzymes to render them almost self-digesting. Eating them actually takes strain off your digestive enzymes. If you find you have any troubles getting used to eating more raw vegetables and fruits, chop, purée, or grate them finely using a food processor.

You may also find when you increase the level of raw foods you are eating that you are having more bowel movements than before – maybe two or three a day. This is a good sign: it means that your digestion and elimination processes are working well. Researchers find the same thing among primitive peoples living on a healthy diet of natural unrefined foods and among children raised on the same sort of diet.

Q: How expensive is a raw energy way of eating?

A: Like an ordinary diet it can be either expensive or inexpensive depending on what kind of foods you choose to buy. Obviously, if you are going to munch mangoes for breakfast and use exotic vegetables for your salads, soups and other dishes, it can be pricey. On the other hand, using the fruits and vegetables which are readily available in season, it can be very inexpensive indeed. The best of the living foods – sprouted seeds and grains – are among the most inexpensive foods you can buy anywhere, as well as being of the highest nutritional value. Living the raw energy way can be *considerably* cheaper than living on the diet of processed convenience foods which the majority of people eat these days.

Q: Do I have to eat three meals a day – even if I'm not hungry?
A: No, you don't. But you need to make sure that the foods in each of your meals are properly combined and that you have left plenty of time (four to five hours) after a protein or starch meal for it to be completely digested before you eat anything else. Many people find, after a week or two on the Raw Energy Diet that their appetite decreases dramatically. If this is the case by all means skip a meal or opt for a piece of fruit or a yoghurt drink in its place.

Q: What about organic foods? Do they matter?
A: Yes, they do. Ideally most of the foods you eat on the Raw Energy Diet should be chosen from fresh, organically grown vegetables and fruits. These foods offer the highest complement of nutritional value to an organism. For most people it is just not possible to eat organic foods all the time. So eat them as often as you can.

And make at least one meal a day a living salad full of sprouts. This solves, at least in part, the dilemma about organically grown foods, for if you have grown the sprouts yourself, you *know* that they haven't been subjected to any chemical treatments. A living salad is also an excellent source of top-quality protein, essential fatty acids, and natural sugars. (When seeds are sprouted the starch in them begins to be broken down and turned into natural sugars which are easy to assimilate and provide energy to heighten your mood.) Sprouts are also brimming with life energy. It is this life energy, which is the power raw food has to transform your health, your shape, your energy and your overall good looks. As yet it is little understood by science, scientists are only beginning to measure it. Something that you will have no trouble measuring after a few weeks of Raw Energy Food Combining, however, is your firmer, slimmer shape and the new lease of life which it can bring you.

8
Just Do It!

That is about all there is to know. Now let's look at the 12 basic guidelines for living on the Raw Energy Food Combining Diet. Also included in this section is a quick reference chart on food combining which shows what goes best with what. Look at them often in the beginning. Soon, however, they will become second nature.

1. NEVER MIX CONCENTRATED PROTEINS WITH CONCENTRATED STARCHES

The old days of meat-and-potatoes or fish-and-chips need to be left behind. Concentrated protein foods, such as nuts, seeds, dairy products, eggs and flesh foods need an acid medium for efficient digestion; while concentrated starches, like beans and grains, potatoes, breads, cereals, yams and pumpkins need an alkaline one. When the wrong foods are mixed it delays digestion, tends to produce toxicity in the system and is responsible both for increasing appetite and digestive upsets. What you *can* get away with is the occasional garnish of protein foods or fruit foods – such as sesame seeds or raisins – in a dish to which you would never add them in greater quantity.

2. EAT FRUIT ON ITS OWN

Fruit passes through your digestive system very rapidly and needs little action by digestive enzymes in order to break it down. If you eat fruit at a meal with other foods its digestion and assimilation are slowed drastically and you can get fermentation in the gut causing indigestion, wind and discomfort. Some people even find that fruits eaten this way turn to alcohol in their stomach, affecting mind and mood. If you want to eat fruit with other food then use it as a starter and be sure to leave 20 minutes for its digestion before beginning your second course. Despite this, however, acid fruits can be used together with nuts to create a meal for lunch or supper. Both the acid or sub-acid fruits can also be eaten with cottage cheese. Sweet fruits such as bananas, raisins, dates, figs and prunes should never be put into a salad which has a concentrated protein in it. The one fruit which is rather unique in that it will combine quite well with raw vegetables in salads is apple.

3. EAT ONLY FRUIT FOR BREAKFAST

Breakfast is a fruit meal. You may eat as much as you like (provided you listen carefully to the dictates of your appetite and you masticate even the softest of fruits until the last bit of sweetness is extracted from them). Your liver – the body's most important organ for detoxification – is most active between midnight and midday. Eating fruit (which is virtually self-digesting), unlike taking in starch or protein foods, allows this detoxification process to continue unimpeded. All other foods interfere with it. You may have more fruit mid-morning if you are hungry. But make sure you leave a gap of at least 20 minutes (45 minutes for a banana) before you begin your midday meal. You must leave 4–5 hours after a main starch or protein meal before eating fruit again and do not drink fruit juice between meals (except as a starter, leaving plenty of time before the rest of your meal, or as a mid-morning snack if you wish).

4. MUNCH A SALAD ONCE A DAY

A living salad based on home-grown or store-bought sprouted seeds and grains is the mainstay of the Raw

Energy Food Combining Diet. While it is by no means absolutely essential that you base one of your meals each day on a salad, this is the best possible way to get optimal support for rebuilding cells and tissues, rebalancing biochemical processes, and restoring normal metabolism. Sometimes, of course, this is not possible – for example, when you are having to eat in restaurants all the time – but then you can replace the living salad with a big dish of lightly cooked fresh vegetables, served with a side-dish of grains, a soup or a protein food or simply with a couple of slices of wholegrain bread. But the more often you are able to make a living salad the focus of the meal, the sooner you will reap the rewards of your new lifestyle.

5. CHOOSE THE BEST
This doesn't mean spending lots of money: it means being fussy when you go to the greengrocer and always choosing foods which are fresh, as much as possible whole (such as wholegrains), and eaten as close as possible to their natural state.

6. SHUN OVERPROCESSED AND UNCLEAN FOODS
Chemically fertilised foods or foods which have been excessively processed to alter their natural state are depleted of nutrients. They often contain additives such as artificial colourings and flavourings which are potentially harmful. These include foods such as white breads, sugar, most meats, sweets, coffee and all the ready-in-a-minute convenience foods that fill the shelves of our supermarkets. These are the most polluting of all foods.

7. MAKE STAPLES YOUR SIDE-DISHES
These are the stamina foods. They include wholegrains and cooked vegetables, legumes and dairy products, fresh fish, organic meat, poultry and game. Both delicious and

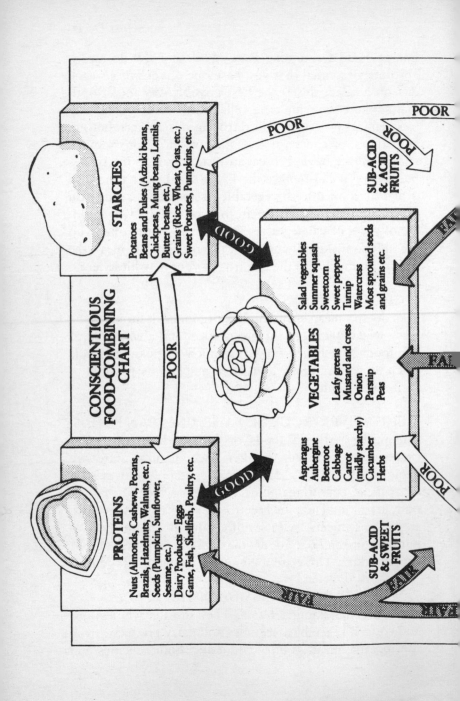

CONSCIENTIOUS FOOD-COMBINING CHART

STARCHES

Potatoes
Beans and Pulses (Adzuki beans, Chickpeas, Mung beans, Lentils, Butter beans, etc.)
Grains (Rice, Wheat, Oats, etc.)
Sweet Potatoes, Pumpkins, etc.

VEGETABLES

Salad vegetables
Summer squash
Sweetcorn
Sweet pepper
Turnip
Watercress
Most sprouted seeds and grains etc.

Leafy greens
Mustard and cress
Onion
Parsnip
Peas

Asparagus
Aubergine
Beetroot
Cabbage
Carrot (mildly starchy)
Cucumber
Herbs

PROTEINS

Nuts (Almonds, Cashews, Pecans, Brazils, Hazelnuts, Walnuts, etc.)
Seeds (Pumpkin, Sunflower, Sesame, etc.)
Dairy Products – Eggs
Game, Fish, Shellfish, Poultry, etc.

SUB-ACID & ACID FRUITS

SUB-ACID & SWEET FRUITS

POOR

POOR

POOR

GOOD

POOR

GOOD

FAIR

FAIR

POOR

FAIR

GOOD

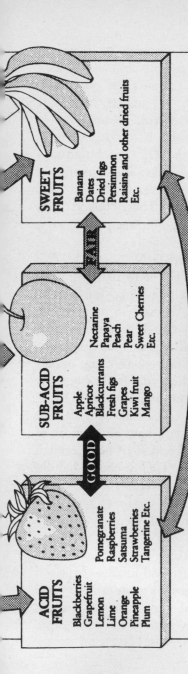

ACID FRUITS

Blackberries
Grapefruit
Lemon
Lime
Orange
Pineapple
Plum

Pomegranate
Raspberries
Satsuma
Strawberries
Tangerine Etc.

SUB-ACID FRUITS

Apple
Apricot
Blackcurrants
Fresh figs
Grapes
Kiwi fruit
Mango

Nectarine
Papaya
Peach
Pear
Sweet Cherries
Etc.

SWEET FRUITS

Banana
Dates
Dried figs
Persimmon
Raisins and other dried fruits
Etc.

GOOD

FAIR

FAIR

FAIR

NEUTRAL FOODS
(they go well with anything)

Avocado   Olives   Seed oils

RECOMMENDATION

All juices can be mixed because they are liquid and can be absorbed by the body within half an hour

MELONS

(eat on their own or leave alone)

Cantaloupe Honeydew Watermelon
Crenshaw Ogen Etc.

RECOMMENDATION

Make meals of one or two combinations, specially of one protein or one starch with one or two vegetables

COMBINATIONS

POOR
Fruit & Starch
Protein & Starch

FAIR
Leafy greens & Acid fruits
Leafy greens & Sub-acid fruits
Protein & Acid fruits

GOOD
Avocado & Acid or Sub-acid fruits
Avocado & Leafy vegetables
Protein & Leafy greens
Starch & Vegetables
Oils & Leafy greens
Oils & Acid or Sub-acid fruits

satisfying, such foods are good sources of sustained caloric energy (particularly the grains) and useful as a provider of proteins for the body's amino-acid pool. They also make a beautiful contrast to the lighter, finer taste and feel of living foods. Use them with pleasure but in moderation. The best way to do this is to serve them as side-dishes at your high-raw meals. This is a brand new and very healthy twist to the traditional practice of making meat and cooked vegetables the focus of a meal which is then eaten with a side-salad. These cooked foods become the side-dishes to the living main recipes.

8. SWIM WITH THE WATER MARGIN

Your body is 70 per cent water. For it to detoxify itself and to encourage the restoration of normal functioning on a cellular level as well as in the system as a whole, 50 to 75 per cent of what you eat each day needs to be chosen from the high-water foods: fresh fruits, sprouts, and vegetables eaten raw. This is probably the easiest guideline of all to keep to, for when you are having only fruit for breakfast and making one meal a day a living salad or supersalad it just about takes care of itself. But there may be days when you find you have eaten more of the staple foods than you should because of being invited out or having to eat in restaurants. Then it can be helpful to make the next day an all-raw day where you have fruit for breakfast as usual, a living salad for lunch, and then another fruit dish or a supersalad for dinner.

9. DON'T EAT BETWEEN MEALS

(Except, that is, between breakfast and lunch – fruit – if you are really hungry). Your digestive system must have time to complete the digestion of a meal before you put anything else into it. Four or five hours need to elapse between lunch and dinner. Otherwise digestion is not complete and increased toxicity can ensue. Do drink as much spring water or herb teas between meals as you like. And if a meal is delayed beyond four or five hours after your last meal you can have a piece of fruit or two to tide you over. Otherwise stick carefully to your meal times.

10. CHOOSE YOUR CONDIMENTS
Read labels on what you buy and make sure that any commercial salad dressings, condiments and seasonings contain no chemical additives, sugar or preservatives. They will only increase the toxicity in your body. Use raw honey for sweetening and then only occasionally and in small quantities.

11. BE CREATIVE
Don't forget, the suggested menus which follow are merely guidelines. Play about with them and make them your own. Figure out ways of getting your favourite foods into your meals. You might be surprised to find just how many of the recipes in the section which follows will appeal to others in your family as well. If you make a living salad for yourself make a little side-salad just like it to go with the chop you may be cooking for your husband. Many a family member has been gently drawn into a healthier way of eating and living by taste alone. Never preach. Have fun with it. If you do it may well eventually turn out to be fun for the rest of your family as well.

12. MAKE TIME FOR EXERCISE
Be good to yourself and make sure that, no matter what kind of mountains you have to move to do it, you set aside a space in your life of at least 30 minutes in a day, four times a week, for exercise – brisk walking is best –

and relaxation. This is an absolute must since it spurs the release of toxicity, firms the body and improves your ability to handle stress. In due course it will become a joy as well. But a little effort is required *now* to make it possible.

Take a close look at the Raw Energy Food Combining chart. Use it like a map to steer you through the new territory of your lean and energetic lifestyle.

THE PRACTICE

9
Go Easy

So you've met the principles of Raw Energy Food Combining, it's now that all the fun begins. For, unlike the usual low-calorie regime with its minute portions of processed foods, the Raw Energy Food Combining diet offers you as much as you want to eat from nature's cornucopia of delights. The beauty and the texture of fresh foods prepared in simple yet attractive ways is, for me, one of the great pleasures of life. When I first began exploring Raw Energy Food Combining for myself, I was amazed to discover three things. Firstly, these foods which were so good for me were also more delicious than any I had eaten before. Secondly, they were simple to prepare. Finally, this way of eating offered such an extraordinary variety of taste, aroma, colour and texture that I was never bored.

All Change

Raw Energy Food Combining is far more than just a programme for weight-loss: it is a lifestyle for high-level well-being – a way of living that will help prevent premature ageing, illness and fatigue. And it is not something which you follow for a period of weeks until you have shed your excess fat, then return to the same old eating habits which caused you the fat problem in the first place. Think of the Raw Energy experience which you will be having in the next few weeks as a transition between the way you *were* living and a better, more energetic and satisfying lifestyle of the future – a lifestyle which will protect you permanently from ever having to deal with a fat problem again. During the next few weeks you will be going through a kind of metamorphosis which will help balance your body's biochemical functioning and put you in harmony with your natural body-cycles. Once this metamorphosis has started, the process of detoxification will continue uninterrupted. And, so long as you continue to make the Raw Energy Food Combining principles the guidelines by which you live, fat-loss will take place automatically – as a natural consequence of the whole process – until your body happily readjusts itself to its most comfortable and natural weight. One of the great blessings of this metamorphosis is that, the further along you are in the change process, the more energy and initiative you will find you have to continue. It is rather like getting yourself into the opposite of a vicious circle: each positive thing that you do reinforces yet further positive change.

One Man's Meat

Here you will find recipes for soups, salads, dips and dressings, vegetable dishes and all the other basic dishes which fit easily into the raw energy way of living. You will not, however, find recipes for fish, poultry, game, seafood and eggs – for two reasons. First, most people already know how to prepare these foods. Second, although they are foods which you should by all means eat and enjoy if you want to, they are in no way *essential* to the transformation which will be taking place within the next few weeks. Indeed, eating too many flesh foods or eating them too often may interfere with the detoxification process. However, if you enjoy them by all means eat them – but make sure that they are prepared simply, without the addition of starch-based sauces, and make sure you eat only one flesh food at a meal. The best way to prepare flesh foods is, as I say, simply – by grilling, baking or poaching. Free-range eggs can be made into delicious omelets or hard-boiled and then grated and sprinkled on your salads.

You can create your own delicious dishes by combining eggs or flesh foods with light crisp salads and serving them hot or cold. But probably you won't want to eat flesh foods more than three or four times a week. They are very concentrated proteins and also low-water foods. Don't forget that for effective detoxification and efficient fat-loss you need to make sure that 70 per cent of what you eat comes from the high-water foods such as fresh raw fruits and vegetables and sprouts.

The Raw Energy Kitchen

Most of the things you need in order to prepare delicious recipes for your new raw energy lifestyle are things which you probably already have in your kitchen. The one machine I consider essential is a food processor. You can get by without a blender as the food processor can do many of the same things but, if you happen to have one, it too can be useful. When buying either it is most important that you buy good strong machines which will stand up to heavy demands.

A good food processor is a real blessing to a raw energy lifestyle. These machines have many varied and remarkable attachments including, usually, a blade, several graters of different sizes, slicers and shredders. The blade attachment is great for grinding nuts, seeds and wheat and other sprouts, homogenizing vegetables for soups and loaves, and making dressings and dips. In fact, many of these can also be done in the blender, but if they are gooey they tend to get stuck around the blade and you can spend five minutes trying to scrape out your dessert with very little to show for it. The blade of the food processor, by contrast, is removable and easy to scrape, so you lose very little.

The other food-processor attachments are terrific for making salads. You can prepare a splendid raw energy salad in about five minutes with the help of these friends. Experiment with grating, finely slicing and shredding all kinds of vegetables because, believe it or not, vegetables actually taste different depending on how they are cut up!

Keep It Simple

The following are helpful if you don't have a food processor and a lot of other electrical equipment like blenders or juice extractors. However, you may find that using these hand-powered alternatives you are a little limited in the variety of recipes you are able to prepare.

- Food processors: there are several hand-operated types which perform either chopping functions or grating/slicing, etc.; some are rather cheaply made, so keep an eye out for a sturdy one.
- Hand meat/grain grinder or coffee grinder: for mincing grains and grinding seeds and nuts.
- Pestle and mortar: for grinding herbs, spices, etc.
- Hand grater: the box kind with several different facets is best.
- Citrus reamer: the well known 'lemon squeezer'.
- Salad basket: the kind made of wire which you go outside and swing around your head.

In a raw energy lifestyle, the things that matter most are, of course, the foods themselves. And there are so many different ways of preparing them that you can probably turn the lack of a food processor or other equipment to your advantage if you let it push you towards discovering even more creative ways of serving the splendid natural foods which you will be eating.

This book contains scores of recipes for you to sample. I hope that they will serve as inspiration to you to create your own; if you do I would love to hear about them. The recipes are simple and portions in them are loosely defined: most will serve about four people. I encourage you to cut them in half, alter them in any way you fancy to include your own favourite ingredients, and even enlarge them if you wish when you feel particularly hungry and want to eat more. But remember that you must always chew your foods *completely* so that you get every morsel of pleasure you can out of them. Remember, too, that you must stop eating immediately when your appetite signals to you that you've had enough. DO NOT OVEREAT.

Look on the next few weeks as a period of transition, take a deep breath and make the leap into Raw Energy.

Here we go.

10
Shop Hound

Now it is time, with Raw Energy principles in mind, to think about stocking your larder. Many of the foods you will be using on the Raw Energy Food Combining Diet you probably already have. Others can be found in supermarkets, healthfood stores and wholefood emporiums. And, of course, most of the fresh foods are readily available at your supermarket or local greengrocer. The sprouts you will use for your living salads can be bought in some supermarkets and in healthfood stores. But they are so much more delicious if you grow them yourself (see pages 77–82).

The list of fresh wholesome food is very large indeed. It contains over 150 quite common foods and, of course, there are the herbs, the wild salad foods, and the more exotic fruits and nuts which you can get if you want to take the trouble to look for them.

Let's take a closer look at some of the different types of food that are available and the specific foods which you may want to choose from to create a raw energy food combining way of eating for lasting fat-loss.

Fruit Magic

The 'great eliminators', fresh fruits are high in vitamins, minerals and enzymes, all of which help detoxify your system at a rapid rate. The gentle acidity of most fruits can dissolve waste substances in the tissues and help carry them away. Fruit also helps stimulate metabolism. Make at least one meal a day an entirely fruit meal. And for maximum weight-loss it is a good idea to spend at least one day a week detoxifying your body on a single fruit. Probably the best fruit (in a temperate climate like Britain) is the apple. Fruits to choose from include:

apple	mango
apricot	mulberries
banana	nectarine
berries	ogen melon
blackberries	orange
blackcurrants	pawpaw (papaya)
blueberries	peach
cantaloupe melon	pear
cherries	Persian melon
cranberries	persimmon
Crenshaw melon	pineapple
fresh figs	plum
gooseberries	pomegranate
grapefruit	prunes
grapes	raspberries
honeydew melon	redcurrants
kiwi fruit	satsuma
kumquat	strawberries
lemon	tamarind
lime	tangerine
lychees	watermelon

The Yummy Demis

Avocados, tomatoes, peppers and cucumber are actually classified botanically as fruits. However, they are most frequently used as vegetables. In fact, they do combine well with other fruits. You can put avocado together with mango, for instance, or cucumber together with oranges very successfully. These vegetable fruits also combine well with neutral vegetables and with the starchy carbohydrates such as rice, other grains, and potatoes.

The vegetable fruits are best eaten raw. Except for the avocado they tend, like most fruits, to pass through the stomach very quickly. The vegetable fruits are:

avocado	peppers (red, green yellow)
cucumber	tomatoes

Go Live

These foods contain important organic minerals and vitamins. They too help eliminate stored toxicity in the system. Each day you can eat as much raw salad as you like. You can use these foods to supply the necessary minerals such as calcium and iron as well.

Generally speaking, most vegetables mix well, both with concentrated proteins and with concentrated starches. Those which are stored (rather than eaten fresh), however, are very high in starch and should be used only for starch meals. Recommended fresh raw vegetables include:

alfalfa sprouts	cos lettuce
artichokes	dandelion leaves
asparagus	dill
bean sprouts	endive
beans – fresh	fenugreek sprouts
beetroot	garlic
beet greens	green beans
Brussels sprouts	green peas
cabbage	Jerusalem artichoke
carrots	kale
cauliflower	kohlrabi
celery	lamb's lettuce
Chinese leaves	leek
chives	lettuce (all kinds)
collards	marrow
corn-on-the-cob	mung-bean sprouts

mustard greens	scallions (shallots)
mushrooms	spinach
onion	spring onions
okra	sweet potato
parsnip	Swiss chard
parsley	turnip
pumpkin	turnip greens
potatoes	watercress
radish sprouts	yam
radishes	yellow beans
salsify	

Gifts From the Sea

If you have never used the sea vegetables for cooking, this is an ideal time to begin. Not only are they delicious – imparting a wonderful, spicy flavour to soups and salads – they are also the richest source of organic mineral salts in nature, particularly of iodine. Iodine is the mineral which is necessary in order for the thyroid gland to work efficiently. As your thyroid gland is largely responsible for the body's metabolic rate, iodine is very important for fat-loss.

I like to use powdered kelp as a seasoning. You will find it in some of the recipes. In fact, I use it in many more – to add both flavour and minerals to salad dressings, salads, soups and so forth. I am also very fond of nori seaweed, which comes in long thin sheets. It is a delicious snack food which you can eat along with a salad or at the beginning of the meal: it has a beautiful, crisp flavour. I like to toast it very, very quickly by putting it under a grill for no more than 10 or 15 seconds. It is also delicious raw.

Get to know some of the sea vegetables and begin to make use of them. Your nails and hair will be strengthened by the full range of minerals and trace elements such as selenium, calcium, iodine, boron, potassium, magnesium, iron and others, which are not always found in great quantities in our ordinary garden vegetables. So will the rest of your body.

You can use nori seaweed to wrap around everything from a sprout salad to cooked grains in order to make little pieces of vegetarian *sushi*. It's often a good idea to soak some of the other sea vegetables such as dulse, arrame and hiziki for a few minutes in enough tepid water to cover. This softens them so that they can be easily chopped to be put into salads or added to soups. Sea vegetables are available in healthfood stores and in oriental food shops. Recommended ones are:

arrame	kelp	nori
dulse	kombu	wakami
hiziki	laver bread	

About to Sprout

The sprouted seeds, grains and legumes are truly life-generating and are the very basis of the diet. These foods contain life- and health-enhancing energies which appear to potentialize and mobilize dormant life forces in the animal organism eating them. At least one meal a day should consist of a large dish of raw foods. This can be a large soup or a salad containing the sprouted seeds and the grains or both. See the sprouting chart on page 86. Recommended ones include:

adzuki (aduki)	curly cress	sesame
alfalfa	lentil	sunflower seeds
buckwheat	mung	triticale
chickpea	mustard seeds	watercress
cress	radish	wheat

Go Nutty

These living foods are very concentrated sources of body-building protein and are also rich in natural oils. They should be eaten regularly as part of the diet but never in great quantities. They are more difficult to digest than fresh fruits and vegetables and are often best used chopped very finely and sprinkled on to salads. When you're eating nuts or seeds at any meal it is often best not to eat other concentrated foods at the same meal. Try these:

almonds	hazelnuts	pumpkin seeds
brazils	marrow seeds	sesame seedss
caraway seeds	pecans	sunflower seeds
cashews	pine kernels	walnuts
coconuts	poppy seeds	

You will notice that peanuts (groundnuts) are not listed here. This is because they are in fact legumes and not nuts at all. They are an excellent source of vitamin B3 and biotin but are also very acid-forming. They should be treated as a concentrated protein and eaten only in small quantities, always raw, never roasted and never heavily salted.

Staffs of Life

Grains were the first food which man cultivated, and they have formed a major staple ever since. They are not strongly eliminative but they are well-balanced foods which contain the nutrients needed for good health – particularly the B-complex vitamins. Wholegrains are also an excellent source of fibre and of sustainable energy. They are important foods for athletes and for very active people.

On the Raw Energy Food Combining Diet you can include your 'quota' of grains by preparing side-dishes such as millet, brown rice, buckwheat (a seed rather than a grain but often classified together with the grains) or wholemeal pasta to go with your vegetables and salads. Or you can eat a slice or two of any good wholegrain bread with your neutral or starch meal. Most slimmers find that they are better off eating rye or pumpernickel breads – the European darker, heavier, natural breads – than the usual wholewheat. This is because wheat contains a high percentage of gluten which in many people tends to clog the intestines. Despite its quite high bran content, wholemeal bread can cause intestinal discomfort which can lead to excess appetite and also, surprisingly, to constipation in some people. There are also some excellent grain breads and crackers on the market which you can buy.

The grains themselves make wonderful additions to starch soups or may be cooked on their own as a side-dish.

Recommended breads and biscuits include:

wholegrain pitta bread	rye crisp
pumpernickel bread	100 per cent rye
home-made bran muffins	Scottish oatcakes
wholecorn tortillas	wholegrain chapatis
wholegrain bagels	

Recommended grains and grain products include:

barley	kasha
bulgar wheat	millet
corn meal	pasta (wholegrain)
couscous	rice (brown)

Take Your Pulse

The legumes/pulses are unusual foods in nature in that many of them are both concentrated starches and proteins. As such (with the exception of lentils) they can be quite difficult for many slimmers to digest. Therefore on the Raw Energy Food Combining Diet few legumes are used – except, of course, in sprouted form. The one which is commonly used unsprouted is the lentil – red, brown, green or black.

Legumes often contain a trypsin inhibitor, a substance which blocks the action of some of the enzymes which break down protein in your body. Because of this, legumes should never be eaten raw, because then a proportion of the valuable amino acids they contain cannot be used. Trypsin inhibitors are destroyed when the legumes are cooked, and sprouting neutralizes the trypsin inhibitors as well. (The sprouting of lentils and other legumes and grains also destroys other harmful substances such as phytic acid [see page 79.])

Tofu – soybean curd – is a very high-protein food which is low in fat and much favoured in the Orient. It can make an interesting addition to a salad dressing or as the basis of a protein salad.

The Dodgy Dairies
Ideally any dairy products that you eat on the diet should be unpasteurized and low in fat. This is becoming extremely difficult in Britain. However, there are some excellent unpasteurized goats' milks available from which you can make goats' yoghurt, and there are some very good simple white cheeses such as ricotta and low-fat cottage cheese; although these are pasteurized they are low in fat and can be used as an adjunct to a living salad or as part of another dish. It's best to stay away from the heavy, hard cheeses: not only are they fairly acidic, they are also very rich in fat.

Free-range eggs, particularly if they are fertilized, are themselves living foods (especially when raw) and

71

certainly have a part to play in the Raw Energy Food Combining Diet. However, they offer the highest utilization of protein of any food. You need to eat very few eggs to benefit from them.

Yoghurt can be an extremely good food on the diet too – particularly if it is home-made (see pages 83–7 for instructions.) Sheep's yoghurt is my favourite. Natural yoghurt helps restore the healthy intestinal flora which have been damaged by eating a diet too high in refined foods or by taking antibiotics or other medication.

Dairy products of note are:

butter (small amounts and best salt-free)
cottage cheese and other low-fat natural white cheeses such as Petite Suisse
cows' yoghurt
feta cheese
free-range eggs (preferably fertilized)
goats' yoghurt
natural/unsweetened yoghurt
sheep's yoghurt

Greet Meat

There is no necessity to eat flesh foods at all on the Raw Energy Food Combining Diet: you will get a full complement of proteins from the mixes of your sprouted seeds and grains, nuts, the occasional egg and low-fat cheese. However, if you do choose to eat flesh foods then they should be those foods which have had the least processing. This excludes most meats, such as beef, lamb and pork, since the flesh of these animals is very high in fat and also tends to contain a high level of chemical contaminants which you want to avoid. So, if you choose to eat flesh foods, opt for free-range poultry, organic meats, game and seafood, all of which are lower in saturated fats and less likely to be contaminated.

One animal-food recipe worth remembering is a Free-Range Omelet stuffed with whatever sprouts you have available; dress with Light Vinaigrette, sprinkle the top with tamari, and serve.

Meat and fish vary tremendously in quality depending upon their freshness and on how much exposure the creatures have had to chemicals, growth hormones, artificial feeds and so forth. You can choose from:

Cornish hens	game
free-range chicken	organic beef, lamb
fish	or pork
free-range turkey	seafood

Sparkle & Spice

Seasonings such as sea-salt, vegetable bouillon powder, tamari, herbs, spices and mustard have an important role to play in the Raw Energy Food Combining Diet. They bring great variety of taste to different sauces, soups, vegetable dishes and salads. Choose the very best and use them in creative ways.

Sauces and Condiments

Honey
Raw honey is honey that has not been heated or thinned. It is rich in certain vitamins, minerals and enzymes, but is a very concentrated food and should therefore be used only in very small quantities.

Miso
A fermented soya-bean paste which is rich in digestive enzymes and high in protein. It can be used for seasoning soups and sauces. It is also a delicious addition to dips for crudites and salad dressings.

Mustard
Either Dijon or Meaux.

Sea-salt
The only type of salt which you should use – and use it *sparingly*.

Tamari
A kind of naturally fermented soy sauce made by fermenting soya beans, wheat and sea-salt. It is a good seasoning for soups, salads and dressings.

Tahini
A paste made from ground sesame seeds which is delicious and very nutritious. It is a protein condiment.

Vegetable Bouillon Powder
An excellent natural seasoning made from vegetables, sea vegetables and sea-salt. It can be used in salad dressings, soups, vegetable dishes – I use it in very many of my recipes instead of salt. It is available from healthfood stores or direct from Marigold Health Foods Ltd, Unit 10, St Pancras Commercial Centre, 63 Pratt Street, London NW1 0BY.

Spices and Herbs

I grow many herbs in my own garden and use them constantly in my sauces, my soups and my salads. However, I also use packaged seasoning, particularly when the fresh herbs and spices are not available. Here are some herbs and spices that I strongly recommend for use in the Raw Energy Food Combining Diet:

allspice	coriander
anise	cumin seeds
basil	curry powder
bay leaves	dill
cardamom	fennel
caraway seeds	ginger (preferably fresh)
cayenne	lovage
celery seeds	mace
chervil	marjoram
cinnamon	mint
cloves	mustardseed

nutmeg	sage
oregano	summer savory
paprika	tarragon
parsley	thyme
pepper (black)	turmeric
rosemary	winter savory

Thirst Quenchers

Juices

If you are lucky enough to have your own centrifugal juice extractor (see pages 432–3) you can make some excellent drinks from vegetables and fruits – for instance, by mixing raw carrot juice and raw apple juice half and half. Building upon this formula you can add a little cucumber or mustard and cress or celery or fresh tomatoes to create some delicious cocktails.

Because these juices contain no fibre the vegetables and fruits mix very well with each other, and they will be absorbed within 15 to 20 minutes of drinking them. They make an excellent beginning to a meal.

If you are not fortunate enough to have a juice extractor you can buy some very good European vegetable and fruit juices which have been processed at low heat. 'Biotta' make several good kinds. In Britain 'Aspell' apple juice is a very good low-heat-processed natural apple juice.

Water

Drink only water that has been filtered, in order to remove some of the chlorine and heavy metals it contains, or bottled spring water.

Tea and coffee

These do not belong on the diet because both of them can leave large quantities of toxic residues in the system. Instead, try Café Hag (decaffeinated), some of the excellent coffee substitutes such as Lane's Dandelion Coffee, or Pioneer, or some of the excellent herb teas. I particularly like those made by 'Celestial Seasoning': my favourites are their Cinnamon and Rose, Sleepytime, Red Zinger and Almond Sunset. You can add a teaspoonful of raw honey for sweetening if you want to.

11
Sprout It

To me, nothing surpasses the best of home-made food. And there are two kinds of foods in the Raw Energy Food Combining Diet which are particularly good when you do it all yourself: sprouts and yoghurt. They are also so simple to make that it seems a shame to buy them. We'll look at each in turn.

Despite all our scientific knowledge, nobody can yet explain exactly how one tiny seed is able to grow into a plant: this is part of the mystery and the power of nature. But the process is something you want to make good use of if you are to rid yourself permanently of unwanted fat. Living foods are unique in nature simply because they have the potential to create new life when germinated.

A major reason why sprouted foods are so helpful for slimming is that they help break through that vicious circle of inertia, which fat people tend to experience, and to replace it with a sense of vitality and energy which makes a lot of hitherto impossible things possible – like feeling positive about yourself or having enough energy to go out for long walks or jogs each day – and enjoy them. Sprouted biogenic foods are able to supply enzymes, minerals and vitamins as well as subtle life energies which encourage metabolic efficiency and provide your body's metabolic pathways with the raw materials needed to function in top form. Just how is by no means completely understood. But what is known about the mysteries and magic of sprouts is enough to leave your head spinning at these little miracles of nature.

Secrets of Sprouting

The most important staple of the raw energy salad, sprouts, are easy to grow any time and just about anywhere. All you need to start your own indoor germinating 'factory' are a few old jars, some pure water, fresh seeds/grains/pulses, and an area of your kitchen or a windowsill which is not absolutely freezing. Sprouts form the basis of living salads, soups and dressings. Most sprouts are neutral foods and can combine with either proteins or starches.

Home-made sprouters

There are two main ways to sprout seeds – in jars and in seed trays. Let's look at the traditional way first, then at the way I find easiest and best.

A simple and cheap sprouter can be anything from a bucket to a polythene bag. The traditional sprouter is a wide-mouthed glass jar. Some people like to make it all neat by covering the jar with a cheesecloth or a nylon or wire mesh and securing it with a rubber band, or using a mason jar with a screw-on rim to keep the cheesecloth in place. But I find the easiest and least fussy way is simply to use open jars and to cover a row of them with a tea-towel to prevent dust and insects from getting in.

Start here

- Put the seed/grain/pulse of your choice, for example, mung, in a large sieve. (For amount to use see the chart on page 86 and remember that most sprouts give a volume about eight times that of the dry seeds/grains/pulses.) Remove any small stones, broken seeds or loose husks and rinse your sprouts well.
- Put the seeds in a jar and cover with a few inches of pure water. Rinsing can be done in tap water, but the initial soak, where the seeds absorb a lot of water to

set their enzymes in action, is best done in spring, filtered or boiled and then cooled water, as the chlorine in tap water can inhibit germination and is also not very good for you.

- Leave your sprouts to soak overnight, or as long as is needed.
- Pour off the soak-water – if none remains then you still have thirsty beans on your hands, so give them more water to absorb. The soak-water is good for watering houseplants. Some people like to use it in soups or drink it straight, but I find it extremely bitter. Also, the soak-water from some beans and grains contains phytates – nature's insecticides, which protect the vulnerable seeds in the soil from invasion by micro-organisms. These phytates interfere with certain biological functions in man including the absorption of many minerals (including zinc, magnesium and calcium), and are therefore best avoided. The soak-water from wheat, however, known as 'rejuvelac', makes a wonderful liquid for preparing fermented cheese and is very good for you.
- Rinse the seeds either by pouring water through the cheesecloth top, swilling it around and pouring it off several times, or by tipping the seeds of the open-topped jars into a large sieve and rinsing them well under the tap before replacing them in the jar. Be sure that they are well drained either way as too much water may cause them to rot. The cheesecloth-covered jars can be left tilted in a dish drainer to allow all the water to run out. Repeat this morning and night for most sprouts. During a very hot spell they may need a midday rinse too.
- Return sprouter to a reasonably warm place. This can be under the sink, in an airing cupboard or just in a corner not too far from a radiator. Sprouts grow fastest

and best without light and in a temperature of about 21°C (70°F).

- After about three to five days, your sprouts will be ready for a dose of chlorophyll if you want to give them one. Alfalfa thrive on a little sunlight after they've grown for two or three days but mung beans, fenugreek and lentils are best off without it. Place them in the sunshine – a sunny windowsill is ideal – and watch them develop little green leaves. Be sure that they are kept moist and that they don't get too hot and roast!

- After a few hours in the sun most sprouts are ready to be eaten. Optimum vitamin content occurs 50–96 hours after germination begins. They should be rinsed and eaten straight away or stored in the refrigerator in an airtight container or sealed polythene bag. Some people dislike the taste of seed hulls such as those that come with mung sprouts. To remove them simply place the sprouts in a bowl and cover with water. Stir the sprouts gently. The seed hulls will float to the top and can be skimmed off with your hand.

Make it big

Now for my favourite and simplified method using seed trays. I find that, with the great demand of my family for living foods, the jar method simply doesn't produce enough. Also, for sprouted seeds, you have to rinse twice a day while tray sprouts need only a splash of water each day. This is a very simple way to grow even very large quantities easily.

Take a few small seed trays (the kind gardeners use to grow seedlings, with fine holes in the bottom for drainage). When germinating very tiny seeds, such as alfalfa, you will need to line your seed tray with damp, plain white kitchen towels. For larger seeds the trays themselves are enough. Place the trays in a larger tray to catch the water that drains from them. Soak the seeds/grains/pulses overnight as in the jar method, then rinse them well and spread them a few layers deep in each of the trays. Spray the seeds with water (by putting them under the tap or by using a spray bottle) and leave in a warm place. Check the seeds each day and spray them again if they seem dry. If the seeds get too wet they will rot, so be careful not to overwater them. Larger seeds such as chickpeas, lentils and mung beans need to be gently turned over with your hand once a day to ensure that the seeds underneath are not suffocated. Alfalfa seeds can be simply sprinkled on damp paper towels and left alone; after four or five days they will have grown into a thick green carpet. Don't forget to put the sprouts in some sunlight for a day or so to develop lots of chlorophyll. When the seeds are ready, harvest them, rinse them well in a sieve and put them in an airtight container or sealed polythene bag until you want them. To make the next batch, rinse the trays well and begin again.

Tips and tricks

Some sprouts are more difficult to grow than others, but usually if seeds fail to germinate at all it is because they are too old and no longer viable. It is always worth buying top-quality seeds because, after removing dead and broken seeds, and taking germinating failures into account, they work out better value than cheaper ones. Also try to avoid seeds treated with insecticide/fungicide mixtures such as those which are sold in gardening shops and some nurseries. Healthfood shops and wholefood emporiums are usually your best bet. At wholefood emporiums you can buy seeds very cheaply for sprouting in bulk. It is fun to experiment with growing all kinds of sprouts from radish seeds to soya beans, but avoid plants whose greens are known to be poisonous such as the deadly nightshade family, potato and tomato seeds. Also avoid kidney beans as they are poisonous raw.

Some of the easiest to begin with are alfalfa seeds, adzuki (aduki) beans, mung beans, lentils, fenugreek seeds, radish seeds, chickpeas and wheat. Others include sunflower seeds, pumpkin seeds, sesame seeds, buckwheat, flax, mint, red clover and triticale. These latter can sometimes be difficult to find or to sprout – the 'seeds' must be in their hulls and the nuts must be really fresh and undamaged. Good luck!

Yoghurt is a Snap

As a health-giving protein food, yoghurt is most important for its action on the intestinal flora. The lactic-acid bacteria it contains synthesize B vitamins, which are needed in the intestines. The acid medium they create in the colon is unfavourable for the growth of pathogenic and putrefactive bacteria. In fact, laboratory studies show that many pathogens, such as those causing typhoid fever, dysentery and diphtheria lose their virulence when placed in yoghurt and are killed even in yoghurt whey. This is one of the reasons why yoghurt is very good for curing gastro-intestinal disorders. It is also useful in restoring the digestive tract after the use of antibiotics, which destroy all the intestinal bacteria (including the friendly ones) plus many of the B vitamins.

Yoghurt is far more easily digested than milk. One reason is that the milk protein in it has been partially broken down by the bacteria. Perhaps even more important is the breakdown of lactose (milk sugar) to lactic acid which occurs when milk is made into yoghurt. This is of significance because many people (whether they know it or not) have difficulty digesting milk. In adulthood they lose the ability to produce the enzyme lactase so that they can no longer break down lactose; this results in lactose intolerance. Undigested lactose remains in the intestines and attracts water. It can cause bloating and excessive flatulence as well as abdominal pains and diarrhoea. But many people who experience difficulties with drinking milk can eat yoghurt without any problem. Another advantage to yoghurt is that the calcium and phosphorus contained in it are much more available for absorption than in milk.

The best yoghurt is made from sheep's or goats' milk. Cows' milk is harder to digest and more mucus-forming. Goats' and sheep's milk and yoghurt can be bought at healthfood shops while plain natural cows'-milk yoghurt can be found in supermarkets.

Make it Scrumptious

Yoghurt-making is really a lot easier than most people think. You don't need fancy yoghurt-makers, thermometers, sterilizing fluids, etc. All you need is some milk, a container, a warm place and a 'starter'.

It is really worthwhile to try making your own yoghurt because, provided you can get good fresh goats' or sheep's milk to make it from – or even powdered skimmed cows' milk – it needn't be heated above body-temperature, and so you retain the health-giving enzymes in the milk. Also, home-made yoghurt is so much tastier than bought. One reason is that manufactured yoghurt is not as fresh as it could be. It also sometimes contains stabilizers and preservatives which prevent it from spoiling too quickly. The result is a slightly tangy sour taste which can put people off yoghurt. The natural home-made kind is actually sweet-tasting. With a little practice you can very quickly become an expert at making it.

Milk

Goats' and sheep's milk are best. You can buy a large quantity frozen and keep it in your freezer if you have the space. Soya milk can also be used. If you want to make cows'-milk yoghurt you can use low-fat skimmed milk powder. This is slightly better than whole milk and is very simple to use as it does not need to be boiled.

Container

Use whatever you happen to have as a container. Either an earthenware pot, crock or casserole, heat-resistant wide-mouthed glass jar, wide-mouthed thermos flask or a stainless-steel cooking pot will do. But it should be made of an inert material: no aluminium or flaky lacquered dishes. The container should have a lid.

A warm place

There are many ways of getting round this one. Country stoves such as Agas are ideal. The container can be stood directly on an upside-down saucer or a wire cooling tray on top if the stove is too hot. An airing cupboard or an oven heated to 120°F (50°C) and then switched off are both good. If you choose a radiator, or the warm area at the top back of the fridge, the container should be wrapped in a blanket or towel for insulation. You can also use a polystyrene bucket or picnic hamper with a lid to make an 'incubator', or even make a simple 'hay box' using a couple of cardboard boxes: one is used as a lid to fit over the other with the yoghurt container in the centre surrounded by blanket/hay/newspaper or any insulating material. The ideal temperature to be maintained is 90–105°F (32–40°C). You can also use a wide-mouthed thermos which will retain the blood heat you need to culture the yoghurt for six to eight hours and is ideal.

Starter

There are two kinds of starter – plain yoghurt or powdered culture (the latter can be found in some healthfood
shops). The yoghurt starter can be of any sort of milk
(cows'-milk if you can't get hold of goats' or sheep's). It
should be plain, natural yoghurt with nothing added.
Read labels! Some things advertised as yoghurt in supermarkets in fact contain no lacto-bacteria at all. And don't
buy fruit yoghurt: it doesn't work and it also contains
sugar. Once you make your first batch of yoghurt you can
use your own yoghurt as a starter indefinitely. In fact, the
yoghurt gets tastier each time you do. If it starts to
become sour then use a fresh starter.

Two Pints of Yoghurt

- Heat two pints (1 litre) of milk to just below boiling
  point (small bubbles should just be appearing at the
  edges of the pan). You can buy a round china disc that
  goes in the bottom of the pan and begins to rattle at
  the point when you need to remove the milk from the
  heat. (If you're using fresh goats' or sheep's milk from
  a good supplier, you can skip this step and just warm
  the milk to body temperature.) You can also use 'soya
  milk' to make yoghurt. In this case you need only heat
  to blood heat before adding the culture.
- Leave the milk to cool to the temperature where you
  can comfortably put a finger into it and keep it there. It
  should feel neither hot nor cold – about blood-heat.
- Rinse your container with boiling water. This sterilizes
  it, which is important because you don't want any
  foreign bacteria in your yoghurt. It also warms it and
  helps keep the milk at a constant temperature while the
  yoghurt is incubating.
- Pour the milk into the container and add your culture.
  You will need a generous tablespoonful of yoghurt for

SPROUT IT

Variety	Soak Time	Dry Measure	Days to Harvest	Sprouting Tip
Alfalfa	Overnight	3 tbsp	4–5	Grow on wet paper towel – place in light for last 24 hours
Chickpea	Up to 24 hours	2 cup	3–4	Needs long soak; renew water twice during soak
Fenugreek	Overnight	½ cup	3–5	Pungent flavour
Lentil	Overnight	1 cup	3–5	Earthy flavour
Mung	Overnight	¾ cup	3–5	Grow in the dark – place in light for last 24 hours

each pint of milk or 'soya milk' you use. If you are using milk powder, mix it with pure blood-heat water in a blender – the more powder you use, the thicker your yoghurt will be – then add your starter.

- Stir the culture in well. This is important to distribute the bacteria – otherwise you can end up with a lump of yoghurt swimming in a dish of milk. (Be sure that whatever you use to stir the mixture has been rinsed in hot water too.)
- Place the lid on the container, or cover with cling film (the yoghurt bacteria are anaerobic). Put the container into your warm place and leave for about six to eight hours. The faster the yoghurt curdles, the sweeter it will be. If it hasn't cultured in this time (it can take up to 10 hours), leave it longer.

Goats'- and sheep's-milk yoghurts tend to be thinner than cows'-milk ones. If you get a rather watery yoghurt first time, don't worry: it is still delicious and it tends to get thicker each time a new batch is cultured. Experiment with the temperature of your warm place. Yoghurt keeps in the refrigerator for up to about a week. Use it with fruit to make delicious yoghurt drinks, or for soups and salad dressings.

12
Breakthrough

Here is a fortnight of menus to get you started. You will find the recipes in the chapters that follow (use the index) – except in the case of the flesh foods. I have given alternatives three or four days a week depending upon whether or not you want to eat the flesh foods. If you do, remember that the best ones are game, fish, seafood organic meats and free-range poultry. If you don't, then simply take the other option. Lunch and supper are interchangeable.

These menus are only guidelines to get you started. Play with them and create your own raw energy foodstyle around what you like best – the best menus are your own!

DAY ONE
Breakfast
Fresh fruit, either *au naturel* or made into a fruit frappé or fruit salad. Have as much as you like but chew it well so that you extract all the goodness and flavour from each bite. If you are hungry you may have another couple of pieces of fruit or a fruit drink mid-morning as well. Should you choose melon as your fruit, don't mix it with other fruits – eat it on its own.

Lunch
Sprouted Lentil Salad
and
Barley Mushroom Soup

Dinner
Green Glory Salad
Baked Leeks and Pecans
or
Grilled Chicken Breast with Lemon
Baked Parsnips

DAY TWO

Breakfast
Same as on day one

Lunch
Red Witch Salad
Yummy Brown Rice

Dinner
Live Avocado and Tomato Soup
Mange-tout and Almond Stir-Fry
Mixed Green Side Salad with French Spice Dressing

DAY THREE

Breakfast
Same as on day one

Lunch
Fresh Orange Juice
(leave 20 minutes before main course)
Bulgar Salad with Endive

Dinner
Gazpacho
Easy Vegetable Curry
or
Curry made with Organic Lamb
Small Sprout Salad with Italian Dressing

DAY FOUR

Breakfast
Same as on day one

Lunch
Green Light Salad
Racy Red Cheese
Avocado Delight Dressing

Dinner
Spicy Shish-Kebab
Kasha *or* Brown Rice
Sliced Tomatoes with Sprout Splendour Dressing

DAY FIVE

Breakfast
Same as on day one

Lunch
Baked Potato Stuffed with Blue Dolphin Salad
Horsey Tomato Dressing
or
Snappy Apple Salad with Cottage Cheese

Dinner
Ruccola Salad
Light Vinaigrette Dressing
Aubergine Paté
or
Poached Salmon with Fresh Parsley and Lemon Juice
Baked Onion

DAY SIX

Breakfast
Same as on day one

Lunch
Celebration Salad
or
Pineapple Treasures Served with Nuts

Dinner
Living Soup
Vegi-Stroganoff

DAY SEVEN

Breakfast
Same as on day one

Lunch
Spring Gardens Salad
Nut Mayonnaise *or* Pink Yoghurt Dressing
or
Berry Muesli

Dinner
Tomato Treasures
Split Pea Soup
or
Braised Vegetables

DAY EIGHT

Breakfast
Same as on day one

Lunch
Greek Delight Plus Salad
or
Summer Red and White Fruit Salad

Dinner
Root-Is-Best Salad
Celery Special Dressing
Free Range Omelet
or
Organic Steak

DAY NINE

Breakfast
Same as on day one

Lunch
Large bowl of crudités served with
Soya Cottage Cheese, Tahini Mayonnaise
or
Raw Houmus

Dinner
Watercress Salad
Italian Dressing
Crunchy Stir-Fry
Millet

DAY TEN

Breakfast
Same as on day one

Lunch
Corn Soup
Cress Special
Horsey Tomato Dressing

Dinner
Charismatic California Salad
(with a sweet Cashew Cream to which you have
added a tablespoonful of raw honey)
or
Ratatouille and Raita Salad

DAY ELEVEN

Breakfast
Same as on day one

Lunch
Courgette Tomato Soup
Branton's Booster
Light Vinaigrette *or* Italian Dressing
or
Organic Lamb Chops
Green Salad with Italian Dressing

Dinner
Small Cress Special Salad
Barley Pilaff
Minty Peas

DAY TWELVE

Breakfast
Same as on day one

Lunch
Crudités served with
Potato Supreme Salad

Dinner
Sliced Cucumbers
Light Vinaigrette
Sesame Stir-Fry
Kasha

DAY THIRTEEN

Breakfast
Same as on day one

Lunch
Greek Delight Plus
or
Stir-Fried Vegetables with Organic Beef

Dinner
Slice of Melon (don't forget the 20 minutes!)
Easy Vegetable Curry
Yummy Brown Rice *or* Millet

DAY FOURTEEN

Breakfast
Same as on day one

Lunch
Scottish Pine Salad

Dinner
Red Witch Salad
Curried Pumpkin Soup
or
Braised Vegetables
or
Prawns grilled in a little oil and garlic

Now that we've looked at some sample menus, let's explore the recipes themselves.

13
Breakfast To Go

Breakfast is sheer bliss; the easiest part of Raw Energy Food Combining. It consists of nothing but fruit. The reason for this is simple: the digestion of fruit is so easy that it demands only a tiny fraction of the energy needed to break down other foods in your body. All fruits – except bananas, dates and dried fruit, which stay in your stomach for about 45 minutes or so – are in your stomach no more than 20 to 30 minutes. There they are broken down so that vitamins and minerals are almost instantly made available for absorption into the bloodstream. And, because they require so little energy for digestion, the energy available to your body is not disturbed when you eat them, so it can continue to focus on the elimination processes which are central to the detoxification of your system and encourage fat-loss.

Fruit Stands Alone

Fruit does not stay in the stomach for very long, it is best eaten on its own. It should certainly not be eaten together with other foods, such as protein foods or most starchy foods – although nuts and low-fat dairy products such as yoghurt and cottage cheese can combine quite well with some fruits. (See the chart on pages 54–5) Neither should you eat fruits immediately after a concentrated protein or starch food. However, when you eat them on an empty stomach – the best way for fruits to be eaten – their effect is extremely positive.

Fruit has the highest water content of any food: between 75 per cent and 90 per cent of all fruit consists

95

of natural mineral water. Raw fruit also contains a beneficient mix of ions (electromagnetically charged particles). This can help enhance metabolic functions on a cellular level and cleanse even long-standing residues from your tissues and encourage weight-loss.

These are some of the reasons to begin each day with fruit. This can either be fruit in its simple original form – an apple or two, fresh berries, apricots or melon – or it can entail using fruits to create delicious and even elaborate fruit dishes to delight your aesthetic senses. The practical advantages of eating fruits on their own are obvious. Breakfast takes almost no time at all and certainly no preparation if it consists of something as simple as a handful of apricots or a couple of figs, an apple or two or half a grapefruit. For most people this will suffice. But when you begin to explore the different delicious possibilities of dishes that can be made from fruit they can seem too tempting to resist preparing them – especially for beautiful Sunday breakfasts in bed!

Detox Dramas

It is not only because they require little digestion, so that the energy otherwise used to digest food can be used to continue the detoxification process, and because they help heighten the micro-electrical potentials of cell tissues that fruits are so efficient for cleansing the body. They are also good detoxifiers because they contain a high percentage of carbon. The high carbon content of fruits encourages them to act as incinerators of waste matter in the digestive system as well as in the bloodstream, the internal organs, the skin and, on a cellular level, elsewhere throughout your body.

Fresh fruits are also alkalinizing to the system – even the 'acid' fruits. This is very important for your body since it can encourage cellular repair and help counteract the acidic wastes eliminated from the cells which tend to build up when you are under stress (most of the byprod-ucts of stress are acidic). Not just raw fruits but also raw and cooked vegetables, help increase your resistance to stress and fatigue thanks to their ability to render the blood slightly more alkaline.

A few people claim that fresh fruit is difficult for them to digest. This should not be the case provided you never eat it *with* any other kind of food or *following* anything else. Occasionally someone will experience a sense of bloating and wind if they are not used to eating fresh fruits when, at first, they begin eating them for breakfast. This is because the fruits' powerful cleansing ability encourages rapid elimination of toxicity, and in the process can tem-porarily create wind and bloating (it can also be because of a severe candida albicans infection). But this is not a com-mon experience. When it does occur it usually clears up within a day or two. If it does not you should consult a qualified nutritionist or a doctor trained in nutrition.

Eat Your Fill

Every morning choose whatever fruit appeals to you and eat as much of it as you feel comfortable with. You need not worry about the calories that your fruit contains. Simply listen to your own 'inner voice' to tell you when you've had enough and stop there. And remember to chew each bite of the fruit you eat thoroughly. This com-plete chewing is the only way you will derive the full ben-efit from whatever you're eating.

Above all *don't let yourself overeat* . . . but don't let yourself undereat either. Eat enough fruit that you feel satisfied. Be pleased with what you're eating, enjoy it, and remember that the fruits you're eating are playing an important part in the detoxification process that will allow you to lose excess fat permanently. If in the middle of the morning you find that you feel hungry again, by all means have another piece of fruit – or even two.

Remember, though, to leave at least 30 minutes after eating a piece of fruit before you begin your lunch.

The lists of fruits you can choose from is a long one – just look at the list on page 65. The dried fruits, such as figs, peaches, coconut, pears, pineapple, prunes, apricots, raisins, sultanas and apples are too concentrated for slimmers (remember the 70 per cent rule): they are best left alone until you have achieved the desired fat-loss: then you can incorporate them into your diet.

Occasionally you can turn your fruits into fresh fruit juices, although it is far better to take the fruit as a whole since the natural fibre in fruit also plays an important part in the detoxification process. A delightful way of getting the best of both worlds is to mix a particular fruit, say a mango, in a blender together with a little orange or apple juice. It makes an absolutely delicious fresh fruit frappé which you can either drink or make thick enough to eat with a spoon. Such a drink is a meal in itself – as are many of the fruit dishes you'll find on pages 99–109. They make delightful total-meal recipes which are particularly good for light suppers. Use them often. Meanwhile, here are the important points about fruit breakfasts.

The Breakfast Guide

- Eat as much fruit as you like up to one pound at a time, but make sure that you chew it very thoroughly.
- If you are hungry in the middle of the morning have another piece or two of fruit.
- Steer clear of the dried fruits until you have eliminated all the excess fat you want to shed.
- Eat bananas only if they are very ripe and you are very hungry and feel that you want a heavier food, and remember that they take longer to digest: allow 45 minutes after eating a banana before eating your lunch.
- *Never overeat* . . . but likewise never undereat. Eat just as much as you need to feel satisfied.

14
Get Fruity

Among the greatest pleasures of Raw Energy Food Combining are some of the beautiful fruit dishes you can prepare as total meals. An all-fruit meal is a wonderful way to end the day – an ideal light supper. Also, a fruit salad with a little fresh yoghurt makes an energizing lunch, and I love making a quick fruit frappé instead of a meal in the middle of Summer when everyone longs for something cool and frothy. Here you will find some of my family's favourite fruit treats. Some are suitable for breakfast since they are made of fruit only; others are designed as lunch or dinner dishes.

These are only my personal inventions. Fruits offer such a wide range of colours, textures and flavours, and there are so many ways of using them, that you will no doubt create even more beautiful dishes on your own. When you do I would love to hear about them!

Remember that you can always start your lunch or dinner with a simple all-fruit appetizer such as a piece of cold melon or a bunch of sweet grapes, or a glass of freshly pressed fruit and vegetable juice. But, if you do, allow 20 to 30 minutes before beginning your next course.

In all the recipes used in this book, C = cupful; tbsp = tablespoonful; tsp = teaspoonful

Tropical Delight
I have an absolute passion for tropical fruit – I think I could live on it! This is a particularly tasty combination of some of my favourites.

1 papaw, peeled, seeded and sliced
2 ripe bananas, sliced lengthways twice then chopped
  into small pieces
1 mango, peeled and diced
¼ C apple juice
30 ml (2 tbsp) coconut flakes
dash of nutmeg

Put the fruits into a bowl. Add the apple juice (you may use concentrated apple juice with a little spring water added if you prefer) by pouring over the fruit. Serve immediately garnished with coconut flakes and sprinkled with nutmeg.

Tropical Promise

A simple yet delicious dish which I enjoy when papaws are readily available.

2 bananas
2 small papaws, peeled and seeded
45 ml (3 tbsp) desiccated coconut flakes
30 ml (2 tbsp) raisins which have been soaked in water
  for a few hours

Slice bananas and papaws and arrange on a salad plate. Sprinkle with coconut flakes and raisins. Serve immediately.

Summer Red-and-White Fruit Salad

A stunningly beautiful fruit salad which makes a luscious full-fruit meal.

1 C cherries, pitted and halved
1 C plums, pitted and quartered
1 C raspberries
outer leaves of a lettuce
375 g (12 oz) low-fat cottage cheese

½ pineapple (outer skin cut off, flesh cut into rings, core removed)
15 ml (1 tbsp) finely chopped pineapple mint or apple mint

Combine the cherries, plums and raspberries and mix well. Arrange a few lettuce leaves on a plate and lay pineapple rings on top. Place a scoop of cottage cheese in the centre of the ring and pour the other fruit mixture over the top and sprinkle with fresh mint.

Spiked Apricot Supreme

Another delicious fruit meal – not a breakfast dish – is this delightful and spicy combination of apricots, coconut and cinnamon.

6–8 ripe apricots, pitted and cut into small pieces
1 ml (¼ tsp) cinnamon
1 ml (¼ tsp) allspice
15 ml (1 tbsp) raw honey

For the Sauce
¾ C dried coconut
a little spring water
5 ml (1 tsp) honey
5 ml (1 tsp) fresh vanilla essence

Blend half of the chopped apricots in a blender to which you add the cinnamon, allspice and honey. Arrange the rest of the apricots in glass dishes and pour the apricot spice mixture over them. To make coconut cream, mix the dried coconut (make sure you do not buy the kind that has sugar added to it) with enough spring water in a blender to get the consistency of heavy cream. Add the honey and vanilla essence and continue to mix. Spoon the coconut cream on to the apricot dish and serve immediately.

Poire Suprême

Who would ever have thought such a splendid dish could be concocted from the simple pear?

4 pears, cored and sliced thinly but not peeled
30 ml (2 tbsp) raw honey
juice of 2 lemons
3 drops of oil of peppermint
½ C blackcurrants

Place the thinly sliced pears in a dish. Combine the honey, lemon juice and oil of peppermint in a glass and mix well with a spoon. Pour over the pears. Chill in a refrigerator for 30 minutes, then garnish with blackcurrants and serve immediately.

Charismatic California Salad

A sunshine spectacular of the acid fruits, with avocado used as a source of protein and essential fatty acids. You can make this salad in any size – small if you want a small snack meal or very large indeed to create a large and extremely filling fruit meal.

1 orange
1 satsuma or tangerine
1 pink grapefruit
1 ripe avocado
3 or 4 large leaves from the outside of a lettuce
15 ml (1 tbsp) lemon juice
a few strawberries (optional)

Peel, remove the seeds and section the citrus fruits and cut the segments into bite-size pieces. Peel and chop the avocado and strawberries (if desired) and mix together with the other fruits. Add lemon juice and toss gently. Line a bowl with lettuce leaves and place mixed salad in the centre. Serve immediately.

Snappy Apple Salad

This is a simple and pleasant fruit salad based upon apples and grapes. It can be served as a main meal either with nuts, such as pecans, almonds or hazels and a scoop of low-fat cottage cheese or a dish of fresh yoghurt. I particularly like it with sheep's yoghurt as a light supper.

3 sweet apples, chopped
1 orange, peeled, sectioned and cut into bite-size pieces
1 satsuma or tangerine, peeled, sectioned and cut into
  bite-size pieces
1 C fresh green grapes
2.5 ml (½ tsp) allspice
pinch of cinnamon
125 g (4 oz) nuts or low-fat cottage cheese or yoghurt

Combine all the fruits and spices. Mix and allow to chill in a refrigerator for 15–30 minutes. Serve the fruit in a large flat dish and top with yoghurt, low-fat cottage cheese or chopped nuts. Serve immediately.

Pineapple Treasures

The perfect dish for a splendid Sunday brunch. Pineapple treasures not only look wonderful, their flavourful combination of succulent berries and fresh pineapple almost melts in your mouth.

1 ripe pineapple
1 ripe avocado
1 C fresh raspberries or strawberries or blackberries or
  ⅓ C of each
a little honey (optional)
30 ml (2 tbsp) chopped fresh pineapple mint or
  spearmint
30–45 ml (2–3 tbsp) chopped almonds or hazelnuts or
  cashews (optional)

Cut the pineapple in two lengthwise, scoop out the insides, cutting the pineapple flesh into cubes. Toss it together with the other fresh fruits, including the avocado; you may add a little honey if you wish. Refill the pineapple shells with this fruit salad mixture and garnish with the mint. May be served for breakfast or as a main meal. As a main meal you can sprinkle with two to three tbsp of chopped almonds, hazelnuts or cashews.

Stuffed Avocado

Another unusual and delightful main meal. Avocados combine beautifully with the acid fruits and berries. This dish is a surprise treat to the palate.

1 orange
¼ C each of blackberries or
strawberries or raspberries or all three
1 avocado (stone removed), sliced in half
pinch of freshly grated nutmeg

Chop and mix all fruits together. Fill the avocado boats with the fruit mixture and sprinkle with nutmeg. (Half an avocado is enough for one person.)

Pandora's Persimmon

This is one of the simplest recipes of all with fruit – and one of the most delicious.

2 very ripe persimmons
¾ C desiccated coconut
a little spring water
5 ml (1 tsp) honey
5 ml (1 tsp) pure vanilla essence

Peel the ripe persimmons and blend thoroughly in a blender or food processor. Pour into chilled dishes. Mix the desiccated coconut in a blender with sufficient spring water to get the consistency of thick cream before adding the honey and vanilla essence and blending in well. Spoon the coconut cream on to the persimmon.

Live Apple Sauce

The quality and taste of this apple sauce depend entirely upon the quality of the apples themselves. If you make it with beautiful red apples it turns out to be a gorgeous pink colour. It is a real favourite for children and makes a lovely fruit breakfast or, served with 125 g (4 oz) chopped pecans, can be an excellent fruit meal for later on in the day.

4 apples, cored but not peeled and cut into small pieces
¾ C (more or less) of apple juice
dash of cinnamon or nutmeg or caraway or aniseed
a little raw honey (optional)

Liquefy the chopped apples in enough apple juice to make a medium-thick sauce. Add spices and a little raw honey to sweeten if desired. Serve immediately, lightly sprinkled with cinnamon, nutmeg, caraway or aniseed.

Almond Apple Porridge

Apples, with their remarkable ability to combine well with all sorts of foods which you wouldn't expect, make a wonderful marriage with almonds. Not a breakfast dish, because of the nuts it contains, this recipe nonetheless makes a yummy fruit meal for later on in the day.

4 apples, cored and cut into pieces but not peeled
¼ C finely chopped almonds
juice of 1 lemon
juice of 1 orange
sprinkling of nutmeg

Blend the apples with the other ingredients, keeping aside 5 ml (1 tsp) of the almonds and the nutmeg. When the mixture is fully blended, pour into four dishes and sprinkle with the remaining almonds and the nutmeg. Serve immediately.

WELL COMBINED MUESLIS

To encourage fat-loss it's best for the moment to steer clear of the traditional Birchermuesli because, for some, the combinations of milk products and grains – even though the grains have been soaked to break their sugars down into more simple ones – can be difficult to handle. Once you've lost all the extra fat you want to lose and your system has rebalanced itself, then you can indulge in the pleasures of the traditional Birchermuesli. Here are some suggestions:

Berry Muesli

150–225 g (5–7 oz) berries (blueberries, strawberries,
  blackberries, blackcurrants, raspberries, etc.)
1 banana
15 ml (1 tbsp) finely chopped almonds or pecans or
  cashews
dash of cinnamon

Crush the berries with a fork. Slice the banana. Sprinkle with finely chopped almonds, pecans or cashews. Add a dash of cinnamon and serve immediately.

Other Mixed Fruit Muesli Suggestions

Blackberries and apples
Apples and sultanas
Apples and oranges

Apples and bananas
Plums, peaches and apricots
Strawberries and apples
Blueberries and apples

In each case remove the stones of any stoned fruit and blend in a food processor or chop finely with a knife. Otherwise the instructions are as for Berry Muesli.

Pear Surprise

A delicious fruit-and-nut dish. Not suitable for breakfast but excellent if you desire a fruit meal later on in the day.

4 pears, finely grated
¼ C raw cashews, ground

Fill four sorbet glasses with the finely grated pears and sprinkle each with the ground cashews. Serve immediately.

FRUIT DRINKS THAT MAKE A MEAL

Apricot Lhassi

A fresh fruit frappé with a delightful Eastern flavour.

4–5 fresh apricots, stones removed
juice of 2 small oranges
pinch of coriander

Put ingredients into blender and blend thoroughly. You may add ice if you wish to make a delicious cold summer breakfast.

Pineapple Blackberry Frappé

A fresh fruit frappé with a delightful Eastern flavour.

2 C fresh pineapple chunks
½ C blackberries
juice of ½ a lime (optional)
spring or filtered water (optional)
ice cubes (optional)

Place all the ingredients into a blender and liquidize. This can be thinned using a little spring or filtered water and chilled with an ice cube or two.

Strawberry Cream Shake

Not a breakfast recipe. This shake is a full fruit meal in itself and makes a lovely light supper for hot summer evenings.

½ C fresh cashews
1 C spring or filtered water
½ C strawberries
15 ml (1 tbsp) raw honey
½ C fresh pineapple chunks (optional)

Blend all the ingredients (including the pineapple chunks, if desired) in a food processor or blender and serve in a tall frosted glass. The quantities above make one very large shake.

Apple Raspberry Frappé

2 sweet apples, cored but not peeled, cut into small
    pieces
2.5 ml (½ tsp) finely chopped lemon balm or mint
½ C fresh or frozen raspberries
spring or filtered water (optional)
ice cubes (optional)

Place ingredients in blender and liquidize, adding a little spring or filtered water to thin it if you wish, and ice cubes if you want a chilled dish.

Banana-Coconut-Mint Frappé

Another full fruit meal that is rich and creamy.

2 very ripe bananas
¼ C desiccated or shredded fresh coconut
5 ml (1 tsp) freshly chopped mint leaves
ice cubes (optional)

Blend ingredients together in a food processor or blender and serve. You may add one or two ice cubes to chill.

Creamy Date Delight

2 very ripe bananas
4 fresh dates
15 ml (1 tbsp) shredded coconut
½–1 C sparkling spring water

Blend the bananas, dates and coconut together thoroughly in a blender or food processor, then add the sparkling water and mix gently. Pour into chilled glasses and serve immediately.

15
Living Salads

To most people a salad is a pleasant side dish you use to set off the main course – which is usually meat-based. On the Raw Energy Food Combining Diet everything is turned around. All the salads you will find in this section are meals in their own right. They can be served on their own for lunch or dinner or they can be combined with protein or starch side-dishes – soups, cheeses, breads, grain dishes, fish, chicken, organic meat, egg dishes or game. They can also be made in much smaller quantities as side-salads to go with cooked main courses.

A living salad is one in which the main ingredients are drawn from sprouted seeds, grains and pulses. The other recipes are for salads based on fresh vegetables. And finally, of course, there are the crudités, which make wonderful starters for a meal or, served in greater quantity with a rich dip, dressing or seed cheese, can themselves become a beautiful meal.

The salads here are mostly quite elaborate and meant to be eaten as the centre of a meal. But you can also make some delightful simple salads by taking a root vegetable, such as a grated turnip, carrot or parsnip, and combining it in equal amounts with both a leafy vegetable, such as watercress, lamb's lettuce or Chinese leaf, and a bulb vegetable such as red or green pepper. This is the classic formula for the simple salad and it works every time served with a beautiful dressing (see pages 128–38 for recipes). It is hard to go wrong following this principle, so experiment for yourself.

Eat it Live

The living salad is the epitome of nutritional quality for encouraging fat-loss. It is made from the freshest and tastiest vegetables and sprouted seeds and grains that you can buy – or, far better, grow yourself. Make sure when you are choosing such things as cucumbers, celery and sweet peppers that they are firm and fresh and also that your carrots and broccoli are snappy and crisp.

Living salads can be made either by hand (in which case the vegetables are cut with a sharp knife or grated on a stainless-steel hand grater) or in a food processor. All the ingredients in a living salad are cut into bite-size pieces, except for lettuces and greens which are either broken into pieces or left in larger pieces in order to form a bed for the sprouts.

You can turn most of these salads into a protein meal by adding a protein-based dip or salad dressing. You can turn them into a starch meal by eating them with a good wholegrain bread – preferably rye or pumpernickel, since the gluten in wheat tends to clog the intestines and may interfere with the elimination process – or serving them with wholegrain (sugar-free) Scottish oatcakes, wholegrain crispbread or other wholegrain crackers.

You should treat the recipes listed below only as guidelines. The real pleasure of living cuisine is creating masterpieces of your own out of the simple things which you grow yourself on your windowsill or find in your refrigerator.

The Red Witch Salad (neutral)

The combination of radicchio with lamb's lettuce creates one of my favourite salads.

125 g (4 oz) radicchio (Italian red lettuce) divided into
  leaves
50 g (2 oz) lamb's lettuce
3 sticks of celery, chopped
2 large carrots, grated
1 C fresh mung-bean sprouts
75 g (3 oz) chicory, divided into leaves
1 avocado, peeled and sliced
4 spring onions, chopped finely

For the Dressing
15 ml (1 tbsp) virgin olive oil
15 ml (1 tbsp) lemon or lime juice
5 ml (1 tsp) Meaux mustard
10 ml (2 tsp) chopped fresh basil
black pepper

Keeping out eight radicchio leaves and five leaves of chicory, mix all the salad ingredients together in a bowl. Then mix the ingredients for the dressing together in a screw-top jar by shaking well. Pour the dressing over the salad and toss. Arrange the radicchio and chicory leaves which you have saved in a 'sunburst' around a platter. Serve the rest of the salad in the middle of the leaves.

Sprouted Lentil Salad (neutral)

This salad is a way of transforming the humble lentil into something quite marvellous.

1½ C fresh lentil sprouts
1 large red pepper (seeds removed), diced
125 g (4 oz) broccoli florets
125 g (4 oz) cauliflower florets
175 g (6 oz) button mushrooms, sliced finely

For the Dressing
30 ml (2 tbsp) sesame oil
30 ml (2 tbsp) cider vinegar
15 ml (1 tbsp) freshly grated root ginger
30 ml (2 tbsp) fresh orange juice
5 ml (1 tsp) vegetable bouillon powder or *soy sauce*

Mix the salad ingredients together in a large bowl. Mix the dressing ingredients together in a screw-top jar and shake well. Pour the dressing over the salad and toss. You may garnish this salad with ¼ C of sunflower seeds if you like; this turns it into a protein salad.

A Touch of the Orient (neutral)

This salad has a typically oriental flavour and feel to it. It is pleasant served with slivers of blanched almonds, in which case it turns into a protein meal.

1 C mung-bean sprouts
1 C fenugreek sprouts
1 C adzuki sprouts
1 yellow or *red pepper, seeded and chopped*
1 medium carrot, chopped into ½ in cubes
½ C Chinese leaves, shredded finely
30 ml (2 tbsp) chopped fresh parsley
2 cloves of garlic, chopped very finely
¼ C chopped spring onions
1 C spring or *filtered water*
juice of lemon
45 ml (3 tbsp) tamari
1 avocado, chopped into small cubes
the outside leaves of a cos lettuce

Marinate the sprouts and vegetables (except for the cos leaves and the avocado) in the water, to which you've added the lemon juice and tamari. Put in the refrigerator to chill. Then pour off the water and serve with small cubes of avocado on a bed of cos lettuce leaves, with or without a dressing.

Blue Dolphin Salad (neutral)

This simple living salad can be completely transformed in quality depending upon the kind of dressing you serve it with. Experiment with a seed cheese, a good mayonnaise or a light Italian herbal dressing to see which you like best.

1 C lentil sprouts
1 C fenugreek sprouts
1 C alfalfa sprouts
1 C Chinese leaves, shredded finely
3 carrots, sliced in paper-thin rounds
1 avocado, cubed
4 tomatoes, diced

Mix the ingredients together and toss with your favourite dressing. Serve immediately.

Spring Gardens Salad (neutral)

Another simple living salad, this dish goes particularly well with Racy Red Cheese dressing, Light Vinaigrette or Avocado Delight.

2 C radicchio, torn into small pieces
1 C alfalfa sprouts
1 punnet of mustard and cress
1 C thinly sliced cos lettuce
2 small carrots, washed but not peeled, sliced thinly
1 turnip, sliced thinly into matchsticks
24 black olives, stoned
4 tomatoes, sectioned into quarters
chives or herbs (optional)

Put ingredients (except the tomatoes) into a large bowl and toss with salad dressing of your choice. Place tomato quarters around the side and sprinkle with some chopped chives or fresh herbs if you like.

Branton's Booster (protein)

This protein-based living salad is particularly good when you feel the need for something quite substantial, especially if you are doing a lot of exercise. Thanks to the fact that it contains sprouted sunflower seeds, this is a salad that really feels as if it sticks to your ribs.

1 C *sprouted sunflower seeds*
2 C *chopped chicory*
2 C *alfalfa sprouts*
1 C *lentil sprouts* or *mung-bean sprouts*
5 *tomatoes, sliced thinly*
3 *celery stalks, cut lengthways three or four times then*
    chopped crossways finely
2 *green peppers, seeded and chopped*
1½ C *chopped fennel*

Toss all the ingredients together and serve with Horsey Tomato Dressing or Light Vinaigrette.

Cress Special (neutral)

This is an ultra-light salad which contains no oil. The combination of lemon and tamari is quite delightful.

1 C *curled cress, water cress* or *roquette*
1 C *alfalfa sprouts*
½ C *lentil sprouts*
2 *sticks of celery, cut lengthways three or four times then*
    chopped crossways finely
1 *avocado, peeled and cubed*
45 ml (3 tbsp) *tamari*
1 *clove of garlic, finely chopped*
30 ml (2 tbsp) *parsley* or *fresh basil, finely chopped*
juice of 2 lemons

Toss the ingredients into a bowl, sprinkle with the lemon juice and tamari and serve.

The Green Light (neutral)

I like to serve this salad with Creamy Lemon Dressing.

½ C *alfalfa sprouts*
½ C *mung-bean sprouts*
½ C *fenugreek sprouts*
½ C *sunflower-seed sprouts*
½ C *chicory, sliced finely*
½ C *cos lettuce*
4 *spring onions, chopped finely*
4 *tomatoes, chopped*
1 *courgette, sliced finely*
2 *stalks of celery, cut lengthways three or four times then chopped crossways finely*
1 *large beetroot, grated finely*
2 *large carrots, grated finely*

Mix all the ingredients (except the grated carrots and beetroot) in a bowl and toss with salad dressing. Arrange the carrots and the beetroot separately around the rim to decorate. Serve immediately.

CRUDITÉS

One of my favourite hors d'oeuvres or salads is a platter of crudités – crunchy raw vegetables and fruit sliced or chopped so that you can pick the pieces up with your fingers. They can be eaten dipped into sauce (see pages 128–38) or simply sprinkled with a light dressing and a few toasted fennel or caraway seeds. The important thing is how you prepare them.

Sticks and Matchsticks

Make sticks from carrots, turnips, courgettes, cucumbers, celery and pineapple. To make matchsticks just keep chopping until you get 'baby sticks' that are about the size of a match (you can also make matchsticks from green and red peppers). To keep sticks fresh, put them into a bowl of cold water with a squeeze of lemon and refrigerate them.

Slices

Some vegetables are particularly nice sliced diagonally. This makes larger pieces for better 'dunkers'. Try diagonal slices of cucumber, carrot and white radish. Very thin slices of small beetroot, Jerusalem artichoke, kohlrabi and turnip are also nice. Large apples sliced crossways can be used as 'bread' for open-air sandwiches. Sweet peppers cut crossways make attractive rings. Try cutting ½ inch slices of peppers and placing around a bundle of carrot or celery sticks.

Whole Vegetables

Button mushrooms with their stalks on, whole baby carrots, the small centre stalks from a head of celery, whole young green beans that have been topped and tailed, florets of cauliflower, radishes, young spring onions – simply trimmed and rinsed, they all make great crudités.

Wedges

Wedges of tomato, chicory, Webb's Wonder lettuce, oranges, tangerines, apples and pears.

It is nice to garnish a plate of crudités with some half-slices of lemon, sprigs of watercress, parsley or mint and some of your favourite sprouts.

SUPERSALADS

Greek Delight Plus (protein)

A new twist on a classic Greek salad, with extra protein added in the form of feta cheese.

4 inch piece of cucumber
125–250 g (4–8 oz) feta cheese
250 g (8 oz) tomatoes
1 dozen black olives
3 C fresh alfalfa sprouts

For the Dressing
1 clove of garlic, chopped finely
45 ml (3 tbsp) chopped fresh basil
15 ml (1 tbsp) lemon juice
15 ml (1 tbsp) virgin olive oil
black pepper

Chop the cucumber, feta cheese and tomatoes into small pieces. Mix them in a bowl together with the black olives. Mix the dressing ingredients together in a screw-top jar by shaking them. Pour the dressing over the salad and toss. Then arrange on a bed of alfalfa sprouts and serve on a platter.

Spinach Splendour (protein)

This delicious complete-meal salad is set off by a subtle dressing based on dry white wine and walnut oil.

75 g (3 oz) spinach leaves
1½ C alfalfa sprouts
6 to 8 radishes, sliced finely
125 g (4 oz) mushrooms, sliced finely
4 hard-boiled eggs, either chopped finely or grated

For the Dressing
30 ml (2 tbsp) walnut oil
45 ml (3 tbsp) lemon juice
½ lemon rind grated
15 ml (1 tbsp) freshly grated root ginger
30 ml (2 tbsp) dry white wine
2 cloves of garlic, chopped finely

5 ml (1 tsp) vegetable bouillon powder or *sea salt* or *soy sauce*
black pepper

Wash the spinach leaves and dry them thoroughly in a spinner or in a towel. Combine all the ingredients of the salad together in a large bowl. Mix the ingredients of the dressing together by shaking well in a screw-top jar. Pour dressing over the salad and toss. Add the grated or chopped hard-boiled eggs to the top and serve chilled.

Scottish Pine (protein)
The combination of lamb's lettuce with pine kernels is unbeatable – another top favourite.

250 g (8 oz) tomatoes, diced
6 radishes, sliced finely
6 spring onions, chopped finely
250 g (8 oz) lamb's lettuce
45 ml (3 tbsp) parsley, chopped finely
1 C alfalfa or fenugreek sprouts
75 g (3 oz) pine kernels

For the Dressing
15 ml (1 tbsp) cider vinegar
45 ml (3 tbsp) sunflower oil
1 clove of garlic, chopped finely
5 ml (1 tsp) vegetable bouillon powder or sea salt
5 ml (1 tsp) Meaux mustard
black pepper

Combine the finely chopped ingredients with the lamb's lettuce and the sprouts. Mix the dressing ingredients together in a screw-top bottle and shake well. Pour the dressing over the salad, toss, and garnish with the pine kernels. Serve chilled.

Celeriac Special (protein)

We've grown celeriac in our garden all winter. It is a pleasure to have this crunchy, delicately flavoured organic root as part of almost any salad.

4 medium celeriac, grated finely
2 medium carrots, scrubbed but not peeled, grated finely
125 g (4 oz) chopped pecans
10 chives, leaves chopped very finely
½ red pepper, seeded and chopped finely
½ green pepper, seeded and chopped finely
mayonnaise for dressing (see pages 128–31)
12 black olives, stones removed
outer leaves from a head of radicchio or chicory

Mix all the ingredients except the olives and the leaves together, dressed with a good mayonnaise. Arrange on a bed of chicory or radicchio leaves, decorate with the olives, and serve immediately.

Raita (protein)

A delicious cucumber salad which can be made with a low-fat dairy yoghurt.

3 finely diced carrots
handful of fresh peas
1 large cucumber, sliced lengthways, then crossways, in order to produce slivers each about 1½–2 inches long
1 C low-fat yoghurt
juice of 1 lemon
30 ml (2 tbsp) fresh mint leaves, finely chopped
crisp salad greens

Make sure the carrots, peas and cucumber are chilled thoroughly. Take a little yoghurt to which you have added the finely chopped fresh mint leaves and the lemon juice and pour over the salad, mixing well. Serve on crisp salad greens.

Devil's Delight (neutral)

Raw beetroot has remarkable properties for detoxification; it's also an excellent source of vitamin C and a number of important minerals. And it is delicious – particularly married with fresh apples. Once you taste it you will wonder how you could ever eat this beautiful red root vegetable cooked.

3 raw beetroot
3 green apples
3 white radishes

For the Dressing
30 ml (2 tbsp) sunflower oil
15 ml (1 tbsp) lemon juice
5 ml (1 tsp) Meaux mustard
45 ml (3 tbsp) chopped parsley
4 spring onions, chopped
finely ground black pepper
5 ml (1 tsp) vegetable bouillon powder

Grate the beetroot, apples and radishes, preferably in a food processor, then mix together in a bowl. Put the dressing ingredients in a screw-top jar and shake. Pour your dressing over the salad and toss.

Green Glory (neutral)

This is a delightful, crunchy summer salad which goes equally well garnished with chopped eggs as a protein meal, or served with a baked potato or a starchy soup as a starch meal.

250 g (8 oz) Chinese leaves, shredded finely
1 green pepper (seeds removed), chopped
45 ml (3 tbsp) lovage leaves, chopped finely or fresh
   mint, chopped finely
4 sticks of celery, cut lengthways three or four times, then
   chopped crossways finely
3 spring onions, sliced diagonally

For the Dressing
60 ml (4 tbsp) mayonnaise
30 ml (2 tbsp) orange juice
grated rind from ½ orange
30 ml (2 tbsp) chopped parsley
5 ml (1 tsp) vegetable bouillon powder or *sea salt*
2 cloves of garlic, chopped finely

Shred, chop and prepare the vegetables and put them into a large bowl. Mix dressing ingredients in a screw-top jar and shake well. Pour the dressing over the salad and toss. Garnish with lovage leaves or fresh mint. Serve chilled.

Tomato Treasures (neutral)

This stuffed tomato salad is delicious and so pretty to serve.

8 tomatoes
1 avocado, peeled and stoned
juice of 2 lemons
2 cloves of garlic, crushed
45 ml (3 tbsp) finely chopped basil
dash of Tabasco sauce to taste
5 ml (1 tsp) vegetable bouillon powder or *sea salt*
2 C fresh alfalfa sprouts
50 g (2 oz) lamb's lettuce
6 spring onions, chopped diagonally

For the Dressing
15 ml (1 tbsp) olive oil
15 ml (1 tbsp) lemon juice
45 ml (3 tbsp) chopped fresh parsley
5 ml (1 tsp) vegetable bouillon powder
1 clove of garlic, chopped finely
15 ml (1 tbsp) chopped fresh basil
black pepper (optional)

Slice the lid from each tomato and remove the insides with a spoon. Mix the insides in a blender or food processor with all the other ingredients except the alfalfa sprouts, the lamb's lettuce and the spring onions; then spoon back into the tomato shells. Toss the salad made out of the alfalfa sprouts, lamb's lettuce and spring onions with the dressing, and season with black pepper if desired. Spread on to a platter and place the tomatoes on top. Serve chilled.

Jerusalem Artichoke Salad (neutral)

A sweet and crunchy winter salad, this dish is another favourite. It is simple to prepare but tastes like something very special.

6 Jerusalem artichokes, grated finely
3 carrots, grated finely
1 apple, chopped finely
45 ml (3 tbsp) parsley, chopped finely
3 stalks of celery, cut lengthways two or three times then
*   chopped crossways finely*
¾ C Chinese leaves, chopped finely

For the Dressing
mayonnaise (see pages 128–31)
cayenne pepper
garlic

Mix together and serve with the dressing. You can turn this salad into an excellent protein salad by sprinkling some pumpkin or sunflower seeds over the top.

Watercress Salad (neutral)

This is a special treat for me because I love the slightly bitter taste and the beautiful dark green colour of fresh watercress.

3 C cos lettuce, torn into small pieces
1 bunch of watercress, cut into ½ inch lengths
4 spring onions, chopped finely
¾ C courgettes, grated
2 carrots, grated
4 tomatoes, quartered
45–60 ml (3–4 tbsp) sunflower seeds (optional)

Combine all the ingredients and serve with a vinaigrette (see page 132–3). This salad can be turned into a beautiful protein dish by sprinkling 45–60 ml (3–4 tbsp) of sunflower seeds on the top.

Root-is-Best Salad (neutral)

This shows how delicious the root vegetable can be.

2 turnips, grated finely
3 fresh parsnips, scrubbed but not peeled, and
grated
2 carrots, scrubbed but not peeled, and grated
1 sweet potato, peeled and grated or 1 potato,
grated
3 spring onions, chopped finely
½ red pepper, deseeded and chopped finely
½ green pepper, deseeded and chopped finely
15 ml (1 tbsp) chopped summer savory or lovage
juice of 1 lemon
2 C Chinese leaves, or lettuce, finely grated or chopped
mayonnaise (see pages 128–31)
spring or filtered water

124

Mix all vegetable ingredients except the Chinese leaves and pour lemon juice over them. Toss well and serve on a bed of finely grated Chinese leaves or lettuce with a good mayonnaise which has been thinned with a little spring or filtered water.

Bulgar Salad with Endive (starch)

A delicious and substantial dish which, thanks to the endive and the bulgar wheat, is high in vitamin E. The contrast between the rich graininess of the Bulgar wheat and the delicate flavour of the endive is most pleasing.

125 g (4 oz) bulgar wheat
1 endive
6 spring onions
a punnet of salad cress

For the Dressing
15 ml (1 tbsp) sunflower oil
15 ml (3 tsp) chopped fresh parsley
juice of ½ lemon
rind of ½ lemon
5 ml (1 tsp) white-wine vinegar
5 ml (1 tsp) vegetable bouillon powder or *sea salt*
black pepper
1 clove of garlic, chopped finely

Soak the bulgar wheat overnight or for at least three hours in enough water to cover. Then drain excess water. Put dressing ingredients in a screw-top jar and mix by shaking well. Add endive, onions and salad cress to the bulgar wheat in a bowl and mix. Pour the dressing over the salad and toss.

Celebration Salad (starch)

This main-dish salad is another beautiful marriage between vegetable and grain, set off by the delicate flavour of sesame oil, lemon and orange which go into the dressing.

175 g (6 oz) long-grain brown rice
3 large carrots, sliced in very thin discs
1 C fenugreek sprouts
¼ cucumber, sliced finely
125 g (4 oz) garden peas
black pepper
1 ml (¼ tsp) vegetable bouillon powder
a few sprigs of mint or lovage

For the Dressing
juice of ½ lemon
juice of ½ orange
10 ml (2 tsp) sesame oil
2.5 ml (½ tsp) grated or ground nutmeg
30 ml (2 tbsp) finely chopped fresh mint

Put the rice into a saucepan. Cover with about 2 inches of water, bring to the boil and simmer for 35 minutes or until tender. Put the dressing ingredients together and shake in a screw-top jar. Pour over the rice while it is still warm and combine carefully. Let the mixture cool completely. Add the vegetables to the rice. Season with a little black pepper and vegetable bouillon powder, garnish with mint or lovage.

Potato Supreme (starch)

This is a light and delicately flavoured potato salad, very different from the stodgy, oily variety which most people know.

450 g (1 lb) potatoes, preferably organic
½ cucumber, diced
5 sticks of celery, diced
2 large carrots, diced
3 spring onions, diced
45 ml (3 tbsp) finely chopped fresh parsley
2 cloves of garlic, chopped finely
5 ml (1 tsp) dill, chopped finely

For the Dressing
75 ml (5 tbsp) mayonnaise (see pages 128–9)
30 ml (2 tbsp) lemon juice
5 ml (1 tsp) Meaux mustard
5 ml (1 tsp) vegetable bouillon powder or soy sauce
black pepper

Scrub the potatoes carefully but do not peel. Add them to a saucepan of boiling water and simmer for 15 to 20 minutes until they are tender. Drain and cool, then dice. Mix the ingredients of the dressing together with a spoon and add to the potatoes. Now chill and when completely chilled add the remaining ingredients and serve.

16
You're the Tops

The fresh vegetables, herbs and other delicacies that you put into a salad are only half the story: the other half is the dressing. So splendid are some of the dressings that you can use on the Raw Energy Food Combining Diet that they will undoubtedly delight your family and friends while at the same time helping you trim away the excess fat.

Dressings come in two varieties: they can be protein in nature, like some of the lovely seed dressings and sunflower creams, or they can be neutral (and used on either protein or starch salads) as is the usual Italian or French dressing to which most people are accustomed.

So filling are some of the protein dressings that they are all the extra protein for a meal which you will need when served with a large delicious salad. Many recipes can be for either a dip or a dressing, depending upon how thick you make them. The dips are best used for crudités; the dressings are best poured over salads which have been grated or chopped or over sprouts.

Mayonnaise (protein)

This is a classic mayonnaise which can be varied by adding different herbs, Dijon mustard, curry powder or garlic to it, depending upon the use to which you want to put it.

2 raw egg yolks at room temperature
5 ml (1 tsp) dry mustard
dash of cayenne

5 ml (1 tsp) vegetable bouillon powder
juice of 1 lemon
2 C salad oil (this can be a mixture of olive oil with
  sesame or sunflower oil or, for a light dressing, it can
  be entirely sunflower or corn oil)

In a food processor or blender, thoroughly blend the egg yolks with the mustard, the cayenne and the vegetable bouillon powder. Add 30 ml (2 tbsp) of lemon juice. While still blending add the oil, a few drops at a time, very slowly until about half the oil has been blended. Finally, beat in the remaining oil, about two tablespoons at a time. This will keep in the refrigerator for five to six days.

Sunny Tomato Special (protein)

A surprising combination of the tangy flavour of tomatoes with the richness of fresh sunflower seeds.

6 fresh tomatoes or 1 tin of tomatoes
1 C sunflower seeds
5 ml (1 tsp) vegetable bouillon powder or soy sauce
1 clove of garlic, finely chopped
juice of 2 lemons
15 ml (1 tbsp) fresh finely chopped parsley or fresh basil
  (if you can't get the fresh herbs you may use much
  smaller quantities of the dried ones)

Put the ingredients together in a blender or food processor and blend thoroughly. If you want a thicker consistency add more sunflower seeds (but remember the dressing will thicken as it stands); if you want a thinner consistency add a little water. Chill thoroughly before use. Made with fresh tomatoes this will keep for two days in the refrigerator; made with tinned tomatoes it will keep for four or five.

Nut Mayonnaise (protein)

A delicious alternative mayonnaise which goes beautifully with crudités and also as a garnish for lightly steamed vegetables.

125 g (4 oz) cashews
1 C spring water
2 cloves of garlic, finely chopped
juice of 1 lemon
5 ml (1 tsp) vegetable bouillon, or sea salt or soy sauce
spring onions, finely chopped

Blend together well in a food processor or blender, chill and serve. This recipe will keep for four or five days covered in the refrigerator.

Soya Cottage Cheese (protein)

Light, high in protein, low in fat and simply yummy.

2 C soybean curd
¾ C nut mayonnaise or tahini mayonnaise or plain
  mayonnaise
5 ml (1 tsp) vegetable bouillon powder or soy sauce or
  sea salt
5 ml (1 tsp) caraway seeds
5 ml (1 tsp) mild curry powder
1 clove of garlic, chopped finely
handful of fresh herbs (mint, lovage, lemon balm) if
  available
30 ml (2 tbsp) chopped chives

Mash the soybean curd well with a fork, add the other ingredients and blend. Chill before serving. This dressing will keep up to a week in the refrigerator.

Raw Houmus (protein)

2 C sprouted chickpeas (sprouted for two to three days)
1 clove of garlic, chopped finely
45 ml (3 tbsp) tahini
juice of 3 lemons
enough water to thin
5 ml (1 tsp) vegetable bouillon powder or 10 ml (2 tsp)
   soy sauce
15 ml (3 tsp) chopped spring onions or chives

Put ingredients (except chives or spring onions) into a
food processor or blender and blend thoroughly. Then
mix in chopped chives or spring onions and chill.
This dressing will keep for two to three days in the refrigerator.

Extralite Tahini Mayonnaise (protein)

This mayonnaise makes a delicious dip for crudités.
Warning: it's *very* rich.

1 C tahini
1 C water
1 clove of garlic, finely chopped
30 ml (2 tbsp) chopped fresh parsley
5 ml (1 tsp) vegetable bouillon powder
juice of 3 lemons

Put ingredients into a blender or food processor or mix
them together by hand until you get a smooth consistency.
Refrigerate. This dressing will keep up to a week in the
refrigerator.

Tahini Mayonnaise (protein)

This mayonnaise is also delicious as a dip for crudités or served over steamed vegetables.

juice of 2 lemons or ¼ C cider vinegar
2.5 ml (½ tsp) vegetable bouillon powder or soy sauce
60 ml (4 tbsp) tahini
½ C water
1 clove of chopped garlic
¼ C olive oil

Mix all ingredients except olive oil in blender or food processor until thoroughly blended. Add olive oil very slowly, as much as you need to thicken. Store in glass jar in refrigerator. Will keep for four to five days.

Sprout Splendour (protein)

1 C alfalfa sprouts
4 sprigs of celery, chopped very finely
5 ml (1 tsp) vegetable bouillon powder or 30 ml (2 tbsp) tamari
¾ C sunflower oil
juice of 2 lemons
15 ml (1 tbsp) finely chopped onion
15 ml (1 tbsp) sesame seeds
5 ml (1 tsp) Dijon mustard

Blend thoroughly and serve on a fresh green salad or use as a dip. Must be eaten same day – does not keep well.

Light Vinaigrette (neutral)

30 ml (2 tbsp) cider vinegar
60 ml (4 tbsp) sesame oil
2.5 ml (½ tsp) Meaux mustard
2.5 ml (½ tsp) tarragon
2.5 ml (½ tsp) chervil
2.5 ml (½ tsp) vegetable bouillon powder or sea salt

Mix the vinegar, oil, mustard, herbs and bouillon powder or salt together and blend well by putting them all into a jar with a screw-top lid and shaking thoroughly.

Celery Special (neutral)

This is a surprisingly fresh and unusually flavoured dressing which goes well with an all-green salad. I particularly like it with lamb's lettuce.

½ C *olive oil*
¼ C *celery seeds*
3 *spring onions, chopped finely*
1 *clove of garlic, chopped finely*
2.5 ml (½ tsp) *marjoram*
10 ml (2 tsp) *fresh parsley, chopped finely*
5 ml (1 tsp) *vegetable bouillon powder* or *a little sea salt*

Blend well by shaking in a screw-top jar.

Horsey Tomato Dressing (neutral)

This is a delightful dressing to serve over finely sliced cucumbers in summertime.

½ C *olive oil*
juice from 2 lemons
2.5 ml (½ tsp) *Dijon mustard*
10 ml (2 tsp) *horseradish*
1 *clove of garlic, crushed*
2 *fresh tomatoes*
2.5 ml (½ tsp) *sesame seeds*
5 ml (1 tsp) *vegetable bouillon powder* or *other seasoning*

Blend well in a blender or food processor and serve chilled.

Parsley Cream (protein)

This is a low-fat salad dressing based on yoghurt. It's particularly good served on salads of sprouts, cucumbers and tomatoes. It also makes a nice addition to a slaw.

1 C natural low-fat yoghurt
juice of 1 lemon
2.5 ml (½ tsp) dill
small onion, chopped
10 ml (2 tsp) chopped parsley
2.5 ml (½ tsp) vegetable bouillon powder or soy sauce

Blend well together by hand or in a blender. Will keep four to five days in a refrigerator.

Pink Yoghurt Dressing (protein)

Not as good as pink champagne, perhaps, but sheer delight on sprouts and cucumber.

1 C thick yoghurt
60 ml (4 tbsp) tomato purée
5 ml (1 tsp) Meaux mustard
½ clove garlic, chopped finely
2.5 ml (½ tsp) vegetable bouillon powder
15 ml (1 tbsp) chopped shallots or spring onions

Mix everything but the shallots together well – in a blender, if possible. Then add the shallots and finish mixing. Serve chilled. Will keep up to five days in the refrigerator.

Green Dream (protein)

This dressing is ideal for a potato salad. It's also delicious on finely sliced tomatoes.

2 cucumbers
3 spring onions, chopped finely

juice of 1 lemon
5 ml (1 tsp) horseradish
2.5 ml (½ tsp) vegetable bouillon powder or *soy sauce*
  or *sea salt1 C natural yoghurt,* or *home made*
  mayonnaise

Blend together in food processor all ingredients except mayonnaise, or yoghurt. Fold into the mayonnaise or yoghurt and chill. Will not keep for more than a day.

Avocado Delight (neutral)

This is a superb dip or dressing, and very rich indeed. Excellent on a sprout salad or as a dip for crudités.

1 avocado, peeled and stoned
juice of 1 lemon
juice of ½ orange
1 small onion, chopped finely
1 clove of garlic, chopped finely
handful of fresh herbs – mint, parsley or *basil*
Black pepper

Blend all the ingredients in a food processor or blender and serve. This dip will not keep for more than one day in a refrigerator.

Creamy Lemon Dressing (protein)

juice of 2 lemons
30 ml (2 tbsp) chopped cashews
2.5 ml (½ tsp) vegetable bouillon powder
½ C sunflower oil

Combine ingredients (except the oil) together in a blender or food processor and blend thoroughly. Then add the oil slowly, drop by drop.

French Spice (neutral)

A pleasant light dressing that seems to complement any salad.

juice of 2 lemons
2 ripe tomatoes
1 clove of garlic
12 chives, chopped finely
5 ml (1 tsp) powdered kelp (optional)
⅓ C sunflower oil
5 ml (1 tsp) cayenne
15 ml (1tbsp) tamari
15 ml (1 tbsp) Dijon mustard
5 ml (1 tsp) vegetable bouillon powder

Blend ingredients together in a food processor or blender until thoroughly mixed. This dressing may be refrigerated and kept for up to four days.

Italian Dressing (neutral)

Another classic dressing. It also goes well with my favourite greens, such as, lamb's lettuce, roquette, American land cress and curly cress served on their own and sprinkled with parsley.

1 pint virgin olive oil
30 ml (2 tbsp) paprika
30 ml (2 tbsp) finely chopped fresh basil
10 ml (2 tsp) vegetable bouillon powder or 30 ml (2 tbsp) of tahini
2.5 ml (½ tsp) dried oregano
pinch of cayenne
pinch of kelp (optional)
¼ C chopped fennel
2.5 ml (½ tsp) finely chopped red pepper

Put ingredients into a screw-top jar and shake vigorously until well mixed. You may thin this dressing with water if it seems too thick. It will keep well for up to 10 days in the refrigerator.

Wild Carrot Dressing (protein)

This dressing is one of my favourites. It goes well either on a salad or on steamed vegetables.

3 large carrots, washed and cut into small pieces
10 chives, chopped finely
5 ml (1 tsp) vegetable bouillon powder
1 C of blanched almonds (preferably soaked overnight in
    1–2 C of spring or filtered water)
10 ml (2 tsp) chopped parsley

Put all ingredients into a food processor or blender and blend with as much water as you need to make the dressing the consistency you want. It's best to leave it thick if you want to use it as a dip, or make it thinner as a dressing to pour over salads.

Green Glory Dressing (protein)

This dressing is an absolute cinch to make if you have fresh herbs in the garden; you may be amazed to find how many herbs and of what different varieties you can use to make it.

30 ml (2 tbsp) virgin olive oil
30 ml (2 tbsp) lemon juice
¾ C fresh natural yoghurt
30–120 ml (2–8 tbsp) fresh herbs from the garden
    (whatever you have available: lovage, mint, apple mint,
    lemon mint, balm, chives, spring onions, etc.)

Place all the ingredients in blender or food processor and blend thoroughly until the dressing turns green. This dressing will keep for four to five days in the refrigerator.

Racy Red Cheese (protein)

This delicious dip or dressing can be served with crudités, over a salad or added to freshly steamed or wok-fried vegetables. It's a beautiful pink colour and has a refreshing zippy taste.

1 C *cashews* or *pine nuts*
1 C *filtered* or *spring water*
5 ml (1 tsp) *vegetable bouillon powder* or *sea salt*
2.5 ml (½ tsp) *caraway seeds*
juice of 2 lemons
½ C *pimentos*
4 *chopped spring onions* or *chives*

Mix all the ingredients (except the chives or spring onions) in a blender or food processor until smooth. Blend in the chives or spring onions by hand and serve. This dip may be kept in the refrigerator for four to five days.

17
Peasant Soups

There was a time when a good soup formed the basis of a main meal for the whole family – and in many parts of the world it still does. I often use the heartier full-bodied soups in this way, particularly in winter. I take whatever vegetables I can find in the garden or in the refrigerator, chop them and put them into a big pot with fresh or dried herbs and perhaps a cereal such as millet, barley, rice or buckwheat. The results are wonderful – particularly if you use vegetable bouillon as your stock. Once you get the hang of it you simply can't help but make a good soup.

The soups in this section fall into two categories – those which are living and therefore either served cold or heated to no more than about 110°F (43°C) in order to preserve the enzymes they contain, and the traditional old-fashioned soups which most of our ancestors lived on. Try both types – as main dishes and as side dishes to go with total-meal salads. I hope you'll like them as much as I and my family do.

Leek and Potato Soup (starch)

This is a delicious and creamy soup which goes beautifully with a neutral salad to make up a whole meal. It is a starch soup.

1 large onion, sliced
3 medium-sized leeks, sliced lengthwise, washed and
*   chopped into fine pieces*
3 large potatoes, peeled and sliced

15 ml (1 tbsp) olive oil
¾ pint spring or *filtered water (more if needed)*
10 ml (2 tsp) vegetable bouillon powder
2.5 ml (½ tsp) freshly grated nutmeg or *ground pepper*

Brown the onion, leeks and potatoes in the olive oil for ten minutes until onion becomes translucent. Boil the water in a kettle and pour over the browned vegetables. Bring to the boil, add the vegetable powder, and simmer for 10–15 minutes. Liquidize in a food processor or blender and serve hot with grated nutmeg (or ground pepper if preferred) sprinkled on top of each bowl.

Barley Mushroom Soup (starch)

A starch soup, this is a beautiful winter meal which is welcoming, warming and friendly. The ideal thing for a cosy winter evening in front of the fire.

½ C barley
2 pints spring or *filtered water*
45 ml (3 tbsp) olive oil
3 cloves of garlic, minced
2 large onions, chopped finely
450 g (1 lb) fresh mushrooms, sliced thinly
15 ml (3 tsp) vegetable bouillon powder
1 avocado
½ C dry white wine
freshly ground black pepper

Cook the barley in half of the water until tender, then add the remaining water. In another pan, sauté the garlic and the onions in the olive oil; when they are softened, add the mushrooms. When everything is tender add to the barley and cook for another 35 minutes. Add the bouillon powder. Mash the avocado with a fork or blend in a blender or food processor and stir into the soup with the dry white wine just before serving. Add a generous grinding of black pepper.

Curried Pumpkin Soup (starch)

This starch soup is charming and spicy and goes beautifully with a sprout salad.

2 medium onions, chopped finely
1 clove of garlic, chopped finely
2 C of fresh pumpkin, cut into small cubes (substitute
  marrow for this if you wish)
30 ml (2 tbsp) olive oil
3 C water or stock
250 g (½ lb) mushrooms, sliced
2.5 ml (½ tsp) ground cumin
2.5 ml (½ tsp) coriander
2.5 ml (½ tsp) cinnamon
2.5 ml (½ tsp) ground ginger
2.5 ml (½ tsp) dry mustard
10 ml (2 tsp) vegetable bouillon powder or sea salt
pinch of cayenne
juice of 2 fresh lemons

Sauté the onions, the garlic, the pumpkin and the mushrooms in olive oil until soft. Add the boiled water and cook for 10 minutes. Add seasonings and cook for another five to ten minutes. Place in a blender or food processor and blend thoroughly. Add freshly squeezed lemon juice and serve.

Bioactive Avocado and Tomato (neutral)

This neutral soup is light and spicy. You can serve it hot or cold.

8 ripe tomatoes
1 ripe avocado
2 spring onions, chopped finely
1 ml (¼ tsp) ground dill seed
pinch of cayenne
1 C spring or filtered water
10 ml (2 tsp) vegetable bouillon powder
5 ml (1 tsp) kelp (optional)
1 green pepper, chopped finely

Blend all ingredients (except the finely chopped green pepper and two of the tomatoes) in a blender or food processor. Heat gently to warm but not above 115°F (46°C). Chop the last two tomatoes and add with the green pepper when you serve.

Chilled Cucumber Soup (protein)

This delightful protein soup 'can't be beat' on a hot summer day.

1 large cucumber
2 C natural yoghurt
60 ml (4 tbsp) finely chopped mint
10 ml (2 tsp) vegetable bouillon powder
1 ml (¼ tsp) crushed poppy seed (optional)
ice (optional)

Chop cucumber and blend in blender or food processor with chilled yoghurt. You may add a few cubes of ice to make it colder if you wish. After blending for two minutes, add vegetable bouillon powder and continue to blend with ice. Finally, add chopped mint and blend again very briefly. Pour into bowls and serve immediately with a little chopped mint or crushed poppy seed sprinkled on top.

Gazpacho (neutral)

Another delicious cold neutral summer soup which you can make as spicy as you like.

6 ripe tomatoes, chopped
½ cucumber, chopped
juice of 1 lemon
10 ml (2 tsp) vegetable bouillon powder
5 ml (1 tsp) kelp (optional)
1 clove garlic, finely chopped
½ red pepper, finely chopped
½ green pepper, finely chopped
4 spring onions, finely chopped
45 ml (3 tbsp) parsley, finely chopped
cayenne pepper to taste

Keeping aside a small portion of the tomatoes and of the chopped cucumber, put the rest of the tomatoes and cucumber, the lemon juice, bouillon powder, kelp (if desired) and garlic in a food processor or blender and liquidize. Add the peppers, spring onions and parsley and mix well, season to taste with cayenne pepper and serve with the tomatoes and cucumber you have kept aside.

Corn Soup (starch)

A starch dish, this soup is uncooked and can either be served cold or warm.

2 fresh ears of corn
300 ml (½ pint) warm spring or filtered water
2 spring onions, chopped
5 ml (1 tsp) vegetable bouillon powder
15 ml (1 tbsp) olive oil
¼ red pepper, chopped
¼ green pepper, chopped
15 ml (1 tbsp) watercress, chopped finely
15 ml (1 tbsp) tahini (optional)

Wash the corn and cut the kernels off the cob with a knife. Mix together with the water, spring onions, olive oil and vegetable bouillon powder, season with tahini (if desired), and blend until creamy in a blender or food processor. Add chopped peppers and watercress to each portion.

Raw Asparagus Soup (protein)

A very special uncooked but heated protein soup, this dish is a delicate marriage of the unusual taste and aroma of the asparagus with the rich sensuous quality of the cashews.

¾ C cashew nuts
3 C spring or filtered water
1 bunch fresh raw asparagus (tips only)
3 sticks celery
10 ml (2 tsp) vegetable bouillon powder
30 ml (2 tbsp) fresh lovage, chopped finely (optional)
30 ml (2 tbsp) minced parsley

Place cashew nuts in food processor with 1°C hot water and blend thoroughly until they have been reduced to a cream. Add to the mixture the other ingredients, saving out the chopped parsley. Heat thoroughly but do not boil. Serve with sprinkling of parsley.

Scottish Barley Soup (starch)

Another starch dish, this is one of my favourite hearty soups. I like it best on chilly autumn evenings. It goes beautifully well with a mixed green salad full of fresh herbs.

1 C barley
1 litre (1¾ pints) spring or filtered water
2 onions chopped
3 carrots, chopped into cubes

6 sticks of celery, diced
125 g (4 oz) mushrooms, chopped (optional)
15 ml (1 tbsp) olive oil
1 tin tomatoes or 6 fresh tomatoes
3 cloves of garlic, chopped finely
30 ml (2 tbsp) parsley, chopped finely

Cook the barley for an hour in the water. In a separate pan, fry the onions, carrots, celery and (if you like) mushrooms in the olive oil. Add to the barley along with the tomatoes and garlic and simmer for 20 minutes. Serve piping hot, sprinkled with fresh parsley. If you prefer a smooth soup, liquidize it in a blender or food processor.

Seductive Celery Cream (protein)

I find this protein soup utterly irresistible, but then I have a special passion for cashews, whose creamy qualities help them marry well with crunchy celery.

1 litre (1¾ pints) spring or filtered water
½ C celery leaves and tops, chopped
¾ C cashews
1 medium onion, chopped finely
2 C chopped celery bottoms
2 medium carrots, diced
1 C fresh or frozen peas (optional)
15 ml (1 tbsp) olive oil
15 ml (3 tsp) vegetable bouillon powder or other
  seasoning

Put into blender half the water, celery tops and leaves and cashews and blend thoroughly. Meanwhile, sauté the onion, celery bottoms, the carrots and peas in the olive oil. Then add together with the vegetable bouillon powder, bring to the boil with the remainder of the water, and simmer for no more than 10 minutes. Serve warm.

High Potassium Broth (starch)

This is an excellent dish to use not only as a soup but also as a broth to drink if you wish to miss a meal or even a whole day's meals, or just as a substitute for tea or coffee during the day. To use the soup as a broth you discard the vegetables. As a soup you drink it vegetables and all. This broth makes an excellent bouillon to use in other soups.

4 medium potatoes (including skins), diced
4 finely diced carrots
3 finely diced celery sticks
2 C green peas
1 large onion, chopped
2 cloves garlic, crushed
discarded leaves from lettuce, cabbage, cauliflower,
    Brussels sprouts, etc.
1 tbsp vegetable bouillon powder
2 litres (3½ pints) spring or filtered water
45 ml (3 tbsp) fresh parsley, finely chopped

Clean and chop the leaves and vegetables, discarding any wilted parts, and put into the pot with all the other ingredients. Bring to the boil and let simmer for two hours, then strain. Garnish with chopped parsley and serve.

Garlic Soup (starch)

This starch soup is for garlic lovers only. My daughter Susannah and I constantly fight over how much garlic should go into soups, salads, sauces and other dishes. I am an enormous garlic fan; Susannah believes that one whiff of garlic is enough to keep her intoxicated for a week. This soup is definitely of my own devising: it is also absolutely delicious. Susannah, alas, has never tasted it. The mere sight of the recipe would make her cringe.

3 potatoes (with skins on)
2 carrots
3 sticks of celery
1 large onion
1 litre spring or filtered water
2 large heads garlic
pinch of oregano
2.5 ml (½ tsp) thyme
pinch of sage
dash of cayenne
30 ml (2 tbsp) fresh parsley, finely chopped
15 ml (1 tbsp) vegetable bouillon powder

Cut potatoes, carrots, celery and onion into cubes and add to water that has been brought to the boil. Break garlic into individual cloves and add these together with the herbs and spices. Add bouillon powder and bring to the boil; simmer for 20 to 30 minutes. Put soup into a blender or food processor and blend, or strain vegetables from it and serve as a clear broth with parsley sprinkled on top.

Courgette Tomato (neutral)

This neutral soup is beautifully light with a delicate Italian flavour to it.

3 medium courgettes, diced
3 sticks of celery, chopped finely
4 spring onions, chopped
1 large carrot, diced
1 clove of garlic, crushed or chopped
15 ml (1 tbsp) olive oil
6 tomatoes, peeled and chopped
15 ml (1 tbsp) fresh basil, chopped finely or 2.5 ml
  (½ tsp) oregano
15 ml (3 tsp) vegetable bouillon powder or other
  seasoning

Sauté all the vegetables (except the tomatoes) and garlic in the olive oil for five minutes. Then add the tomatoes and pour in enough boiling water to cover. Bring to the boil and simmer for 20–30 minutes. Serve sprinkled with fresh basil or oregano and season according to taste.

Split-Pea Soup (starch)

Another hearty starch soup which goes well with a green salad.

1 C dried split peas which have been soaked in water to
  cover overnight
1 large onion, chopped
2 medium carrots, diced
2 sticks of celery, diced
1 litre (1¾ pints) spring or filtered water
15 ml (1 tbsp) vegetable bouillon powder
30 ml (2 tbsp) chopped fresh herbs as available (parsley,
  lovage, sage, pot marjoram)

After the peas have been washed and soaked overnight, put them in a pot with all the vegetables and cover with water. Bring to the boil and simmer for 1½ hours until the peas are tender. Add the vegetable bouillon and fresh herbs five minutes before serving. If you want a smooth soup, put into a food processor or blender; otherwise serve as is.

18
Hot Veggies

Cooked vegetables have a marvellous flavour of their own
– there's nothing like the crunchy pleasure of a baked
potato stuffed with a well dressed living salad, the light
crisp taste of stir-fried mange-tout spiked with almond
slivers, or the spicy tang of a good curry. Each vegetable
has its own character and, like a special child, needs to be
handled in an individual way to get the most from it.

In this section you will find all sorts of vegetable dishes
prepared in many different ways. Some are best used as
small side-dishes; others – particularly some of the mixtures – make wonderful meals in themselves and are great
for entertaining.

SUPER STIR-FRIES

These attractive and quick vegetable dishes are based on
the Chinese principle of frying vegetables very quickly in
a minute quantity of light oil. If you're in a hurry, all of
your vegetables may be prepared in advance, chopped
and left in the refrigerator for when you are ready to
cook them.

Each stir-fry recipe is based upon the same principles
and there are many different combinations you can try.
We stir-fry any vegetables that we can find sitting in the
refrigerator. With larger vegetables such as cauliflower
florets, the trick is to cut them fine enough so that they
can cook within a three minute period. Here are a few
suggestions, but don't be afraid to create your own
combinations.

Mange-tout and Almond Stir-Fry (protein)

A delightful protein dish, thanks to the combination of delicate green mange-tout and crunchy almonds.

250 g (8 oz) mange-tout
30 ml (2 tbsp) soya oil
50 g (2 oz) almonds (preferably blanched)
125 g (4 oz) button mushrooms
5 ml (1 tsp) vegetable bouillon powder

Top and tail the mange-tout. Heat oil in a wok or large frying pan and when hot add the almonds and stir-fry for three to five minutes. Then add the remaining ingredients and continue to stir-fry for another two to three minutes. Serve immediately.

Ultra-High Stir-Fry (neutral)

This neutral recipe is based on the sprouts – whatever sprouts you have will do nicely. Chinese mung-bean sprouts are traditionally used.

10 ml (2 tsp) soya oil
250 g (8 oz) mung sprouts or *other sprouted seeds* or
  grains
black pepper, freshly ground
1 large red pepper, deseeded
5 ml (1 tsp) vegetable bouillon powder or *soy sauce*

Heat the oil in a wok or large frying pan. When hot, stir-fry the sprouts and pepper for one to two minutes. Add a little vegetable bouillon powder or soy sauce, season with black pepper, and serve immediately.

Green Stir-Fry (protein)

A lovely protein dish which goes well with a watercress salad.

15 ml (1 tbsp) soya oil
50 g (2 oz) cashew nuts or cashew-nut pieces
2 cloves garlic, chopped finely
250 g (8 oz) Chinese leaves, shredded
250 g (8 oz) broccoli florets
250 g (8 oz) green beans, sliced diagonally
5 ml (1 tsp) vegetable bouillon powder
15 ml (1 tbsp) spring or filtered water
juice of 1 lemon

Heat the oil in a wok or large frying pan. When hot, stir-fry the cashews and garlic for two to three minutes. Then add the vegetables and stir-fry for a further three to four minutes. Mix the vegetable bouillon powder with the water and lemon juice and pour over the vegetables and nuts and stir in well. Serve immediately.

Sesame-Courgette Stir-Fry (protein)

A light protein recipe which my son Jesse adores.

10 ml (2 tsp) sesame seed oil or soya oil
125 g (4 oz) sesame seeds
250 g (8 oz) courgettes
8 sticks of celery
250 g (8 oz) carrots
5 ml (1 tsp) vegetable bouillon powder or tamari

Cut up the vegetables into matchsticks. Heat the oil in a wok or large frying pan. When hot, add the sesame seeds and cook at a high heat for one to two minutes until they begin to brown. Then add the vegetables and cook for another two to three minutes. Season with bouillon powder or tamari and serve immediately.

Russian Red Stir-Fry (neutral)

A very light refreshing cabbage dish which is quick and easy to prepare.

350 g (¾ lb) red cabbage or *Savoy cabbage*
250 g (½ lb) white turnip
15 ml (1 tbsp) olive oil
4 spring onions, chopped finely
15 ml (1 tbsp) soy sauce
15 ml (1 tbsp) tomato purée
5 ml (1 tsp) cumin seeds
5 ml (1 tsp) paprika
5 ml (1 tsp) vegetable bouillon powder
freshly ground black pepper

Wash the cabbage and shred finely. Grate the turnip finely. Heat the oil in a large saucepan or wok and fry the cabbage–turnip mixture together with the spring onions over a high heat for three minutes. Add the remaining ingredients (including a little spring or filtered water if necessary) and cook for a further five minutes. Season with black pepper and serve immediately.

OTHER FAVOURITE VEGETABLE RECIPES

Artichokes (neutral)

Artichokes are one of my favourite vegetables. I like them served in almost any form. A simple vinaigrette sauce is perhaps best of all.

4 large artichokes
juice of ½ a lemon
sea-salt to taste
vinaigrette sauce or *dip* or *seed milk*

Place the artichokes in a large pot of boiling water – at least 3 inch depth of water. Add the lemon juice and a pinch or two of sea-salt to season, and bring to the boil. Simmer for 45 minutes until the meat at the bottom of each artichoke leaf is softened. Remove and serve either hot or cold with a simple vinaigrette sauce or one of the richer dips or seed milks.

Corn on the Cob (starch)

4 corn-cobs
sea-salt to season
Tahini Mayonnaise dressing (see page 132) or a little
  butter and salt

Remove the corn husks and silk. Place the cobs in boiling, salted water and cook for 10–12 minutes. Strain and serve with Tahini Mayonnaise dressing or a little butter and salt.

Minty Peas (starch)

450 g (1 lb) fresh shelled garden peas
2.5 ml (½ tsp) vegetable bouillon powder
15 ml (1 tbsp) spring or filtered water
30 ml (2 tbsp) fresh mint (apple mint is particularly
  good)

Put the peas into a pot with the water and vegetable bouillon powder and gently steam over a low heat for 15–20 minutes. Sprinkle with the mint for the last five minutes of cooking and serve immediately.

Pumpkin in Tahini (starch)

The small amount of tahini used here does not interfere with this starch vegetable and sets it off nicely.

1 large onion chopped finely
15 ml (1 tbsp) olive oil
15 ml (1 tbsp) tahini
450 g (1 lb) fresh pumpkin (skin removed), cut into 1
  inch cubes
2.5 ml (½ tsp) grated nutmeg

Sauté the onion in the oil until brown, then add the pumpkin and continue to sauté for 5–10 minutes, stirring carefully. Add a splash of water if necessary and leave on a very low heat for another 10–15 minutes until soft. Add the tahini and mix well. Serve immediately sprinkled with the grated nutmeg.

Easy Vegetable Curry (starch)

This takes no more than 20–30 minutes to prepare. It can be eaten on its own or with a light salad for supper. In smaller quantities serve as a side-dish for a living salad.

1 large onion, chopped finely
15 ml (1 tbsp) soya oil or olive oil or sunflower oil
10 ml (2 tsp) mild curry powder
3 large carrots, sliced tlengthways, then cut across to
  make 1½ inch sticks
1 medium-sized turnip, cut up finely into matchsticks
2 potatoes
5–7.5 ml (1–1½ tsp) vegetable bouillon powder
1½ C spring or filtered water
grated coconut (optional)

Sauté the onion in the oil until it becomes translucent, then add the curry powder and vegetable bouillon powder and continue to stir for a few minutes. Add the rest of the vegetables and pour in the water. Bring to the boil and simmer slowly for 20–30 minutes, then serve. It is particularly nice served with some grated dried coconut.

During the summer it's delightful to be able to add some French beans or some peas (I often like to add some chopped celery) – or, really, whatever other vegetables you have in the refrigerator.

Spicy Shish Kebab (neutral)

A delicious marinated, skewered vegetable dish which you can grill or barbecue. Serve it on a bed of brown rice cooked with vegetable bouillon powder and herbs. You will need two skewers for each person and it's a good idea to marinate the vegetables for two to four hours.

1 large aubergine, cut into 1¼ inch chunks
10 fresh tomatoes, halved
24 large mushrooms
1 red pepper
1 green pepper
2 large onions (preferably red), cut into 1 inch chunks
1 large swede or 2 small turnips, cut into 1 inch chunks

For the Marinade
1¼ C olive oil
juice from 3 lemons
30 ml (2 tbsp) red wine
3 cloves of garlic, crushed
5 ml (1 tsp) coriander, crushed
30 ml (2 tbsp) of parsley, finely chopped
2.5 ml (½ tsp) nutmeg, finely ground
15 ml (1 tbsp) fresh basil (optional)
2.5 ml (1 tsp) dried oregano

Wash, cut and prepare the vegetables. Place all the marinade ingredients together in a large bowl and mix thoroughly. Grill the aubergine until just soft and add with the rest of the vegetables to the marinade. Let it all sit for two to four hours. Skewer the vegetables, alternating from one to another, and baste them with the marinade as they are grilled or barbecued. May be served with a spicy sauce such as a tahini sauce, mayonnaise or chili sauce.

Aubergine Paté (protein)

I learned this recipe from a Middle Eastern friend who served it to me once. I had absolutely no idea what I was eating but found it completely irresistible. I have never forgotten the experience. You can vary the taste of it considerably by adding different spices or different extra ingredients.

2 medium aubergines
4 cloves of garlic, finely chopped
60 ml (4 tbsp) fresh parsley, finely chopped
1 small onion, finely chopped
½ C tahini
5 ml (1 tsp) vegetable bouillon powder or *other seasoning*
2.5 ml (½ tsp) ground cumin
pinch of cayenne
15 ml (1 tbsp) olive oil or *Tahini Mayonnaise (see page 132)*

Remove the stems from the aubergines and prick them with a fork as you would a potato. Put them into an oven and bake slowly until they become soft inside. Remove them, then scoop out the insides and put into a food processor to purée. Combine all the other ingredients (except the oil) in the food processor with the purée, remove and chill in a refrigerator. Pour the olive oil on top just before serving. You can use Tahini Mayonnaise instead of the olive oil as a delicious variation.

Vegi-stroganoff (protein)

A splendid protein-based vegetable dish that can be a real success for entertaining.

900–1150 g (2–2½ lb) chopped fresh vegetables (carrots, celery, courgettes, aubergine, cabbage, Chinese leaves, small tomatoes, cauliflower, broccoli, peas, etc.)

For the Sauce
1½ C raw cashews or cashew pieces
1½ C filtered or spring water (more if needed)
250 g (8 oz) chopped mushrooms
1 large onion, chopped finely
15 ml (1 tbsp) soya oil or olive oil
juice of 2 lemons
15 ml (3 tsp) vegetable bouillon powder
black pepper
1 ml (¼ tsp) dill
2.5–5 ml (½–1 tsp) paprika
45 ml (3 tbsp) dry red wine

To make the sauce, mince the cashew nuts finely in a food processor, then add the water and mix further into a creamy consistency. Sauté the mushrooms and onion in the oil until the onion is translucent. Then mix in all remaining sauce ingredients except the red wine. Cook very slowly, either in a double boiler or on a very slow burner. Then steam all the chopped vegetables in a little water. As soon as the vegetables are steamed, which usually takes 20–30 minutes, pour the sauce and wine over them, sprinkle with a dash of paprika and serve immediately.

Ginger Beans (starch)

5 ml (1 tsp) soya or other oil
450 g (1 lb) French beans
2 cloves garlic, chopped finely
15 ml (1 tbsp) fresh ginger, chopped finely
juice of 1 lemon
15 ml (1 tbsp) tamari or soy sauce

Put oil into a wok or large frying pan and heat. When hot, add vegetables, garlic and ginger and stir constantly. Cook for three to four minutes, season with tamari or soy sauce, and serve immediately.

Ratatouille (neutral)

A low-fat recipe which makes a delicious main meal eaten with either a protein or a starch salad. It's very filling.

2 large aubergines
1 large onion
4 cloves of garlic
15 ml (1 tbsp) olive oil
15 ml (1 tbsp) fresh basil or 5 ml (1 tsp) dried basil
450 g (1 lb) fresh skinned tomatoes or 450 g (15 oz) tin
  of tomatoes
1 large green pepper, deseeded and chopped
175 g (6 oz) fresh mushrooms
250 g (½ lb) courgettes, sliced
15 ml (1 tbsp) vegetable bouillon powder
freshly ground black pepper
45 ml (3 tbsp) chopped fresh parsley

Cut the aubergine into ½ inch cubes; chop the onion and the garlic finely. Heat the oil, then brown the aubergine, onion and garlic in the oil for five to ten minutes. Add the basil and cook for one more minute, then add tomatoes, green pepper, mushrooms, courgettes and bouillon powder and simmer for 25 minutes. Season with pepper and sprinkle with parsley. May be served either hot or chilled.

Braised Vegetables (starch)

This simple and inexpensive dish is a favourite with my son Aaron. It combines well with a living salad using a neutral or a starch dressing.

1 head of celery
6 medium potatoes
5 large carrots
2 C spring or filtered water
1 bay leaf
5 ml (1 tsp) vegetable bouillon powder
15 ml (1 tbsp) tahini
freshly ground black pepper

Scrub the vegetables and cut into strips about 3 inches long. Place in a large pot with water, bay leaf and vegetable bouillon powder; put into an oven pre-heated to 400°F (200°C), gas mark 6 and bake for 20 minutes. Add tahini and stir well, then replace in oven for a further five minutes. Season with black pepper and serve at once.

Baked Vegetables

I am extremely fond of baked vegetables because the process of baking seems to help the vegetables maintain their natural flavour. Besides, there is something quite charming to me about serving a whole baked onion at a meal: it's amusing as well as delicious.

Baking vegetables is one of the best methods of preserving their vitamins and minerals. You can bake vegetables either on their own or hidden within wholegrain pastry, or you can mix them together in a kind of hot-pot.

Jacket Potatoes (starch)

Baked potatoes make the most wonderful 'pockets' for salads, stir-fried vegetables, steamed vegetables and so forth. What you need to avoid are the traditional cheese, sour-cream, yoghurt, etc., baked potato fillings because the combination of the starchy potato and the protein of cheese or other dairy products is not a good one. However, there are many neutral vegetables and salads and dips that you can put into baked potatoes, from mashed avocados mixed together with some garlic and a little vegetable bouillon powder to a simple living salad of sprouts with a herbal dressing. One of my most favourite dishes of all is of baked potatoes which have been stuffed with such delicacies.

Pre-heat the oven to 400°F (200°C), gas mark 6. Scrub the potatoes carefully with a natural bristled brush but do not peel. Pierce the skins two or three times with a fork and bake for 1–1½ hours or until soft. Slit the potatoes open and fill with your desired filling – perhaps a little neutral salad dressing or a little mashed avocado and lemon. Baked potatoes are particularly delicious when sprinkled with fresh parsley which has been chopped finely.

Baked Leeks and Pecans (protein)

450 g (1 lb) leeks
15 ml (1 tbsp) soya oil or other cooking oil
125 g (4 oz) pecans
30 ml (2 tbsp) miso
splash of spring or filtered water

Slice the leeks lengthways in very fine strips and then cut into 3 inch lengths. Mix well with the oil and bake in a hot oven for 10–15 minutes. Chop the pecans finely in a food processor and combine with the miso and a little water to prepare a sauce for the leeks. Cover the leeks with the sauce and serve immediately.

Baked Carrots (protein)

6 large healthy carrots
30 ml (1 tbsp) olive oil or soya oil
¼ C sesame seeds

Scrub the carrots well and slice them lengthways four or five times, then crossways into pieces about 3 inches long. Mix well with the oil, then place on a baking sheet and bake in a hot oven for 20 minutes. During the last 10 minutes of baking spread the sesame seeds over the top. Serve immediately.

Baked Parsnips (neutral)

450 g (1 lb) fresh parsnips
15–30 ml (1–2 tbsp) sesame oil or olive oil
2.5 ml (½ tsp) vegetable bouillon powder
30 ml (2 tbsp) Dijon mustard

Slice the parsnips lengthways two or three times, then crossways into lengths about 3 inches long. Mix together the oil, the vegetable bouillon powder and the mustard and pour over to cover the parsnips. Bake in a moderate oven until golden brown – about 30–35 minutes.

Baked Turnips (neutral)

450 g (1 lb) fresh turnips
15–30 ml (1–2 tbsp) oil
5 ml (1 tsp) fresh ginger
2.5 ml (½ tsp) vegetable bouillon powder
45 ml (3 tbsp) spring or filtered water

Cut the turnips into matchstick-sized strips and put into a casserole with the oil, the finely sliced ginger, the vegetable bouillon powder and the water. Cover with a lid and bake in a moderate oven until tender.

Baked Onions (neutral)

4 large Spanish onions
chopped parsley (as garnish)

Top and tail the onions but leave the outer skin on. Bake in a medium oven for 20–30 minutes until they are yielding to the touch. Take from the oven, remove the outer skins and serve immediately with a sprinkling of chopped parsley to garnish.

19
Gorgeous Grains

Six thousand years ago Zarathustra (Zoroaster), the Persian sage, waxed ecstatic about grains: 'When the light of the moon waxeth warmer,' he said, 'golden-hued grains grow up from the earth during the spring.' I think these words beautifully capture the richness and delight of the grain foods. Grains should always be eaten as close as possible to their natural state. The best way of all to eat them is sprouted. The next best is by cooking them slowly and eating them in side-dishes to go with living salads or supersalads.

The grains are rich in B-complex vitamins. And, providing they are unrefined, they are also rich in fibre. They are excellent foods for providing simple, long-sustained energy – as such, grain dishes play an important part in the diet of athletes. The leaner you become the more you will wish to increase the amount of grains you are eating.

Here are a few simple grain recipes to get you started.

Yummy Brown Rice (starch)

Rice cooked in this manner is so delicious that it seems to be a worthwhile dish in itself. It needs no special sauces or condiments to make it work.

1 C brown rice
2–3 C spring or filtered water
15 ml (1 tbsp) olive oil
10 ml (2 tsp) vegetable bouillon powder
15 ml (3 tbsp) fresh parsley, chopped
5 ml (1 tsp) pot marjoram
2 cloves garlic, finely chopped (optional)

Wash the rice three times under running water and put into a saucepan. Boil the water in a kettle and pour over the rice. Add seasonings except for 1 tbsp of the parsley. Bring to the boil and cook gently for 45 minutes or until all the liquid has been absorbed. Garnish with parsley and serve. (You can double this recipe and prepare enough rice to make a large rice salad the next day.)

Kasha (starch)

A favourite of the Russians, kasha is also a favourite of mine. It is quick to cook and has a pleasant nutty flavour.

2 C buckwheat groats
spring or filtered water to cover
10 ml (2 tsp) vegetable bouillon powder
30 ml (2 tbsp) chopped fresh parsley or other herbs

Place buckwheat in a heavy-bottomed pan and roast it dry over a medium heat while stirring with a wooden spoon. As it begins to darken pour hot water over the buckwheat and add the vegetable bouillon powder and 1 tbsp of the herbs. Cover and simmer very slowly for 15–20 minutes until all the liquid has been absorbed. Serve with the remaining herbs sprinkled on the top.

Polenta (starch)

Polenta is a peasant dish made from cornmeal. I particularly like it served with a living salad dressed with a spicy sauce which I put on the polenta as well.

3 C filtered or spring water
1 C cornmeal
10 ml (2 tsp) vegetable bouillon powder or tamari

Heat the water in a kettle. Pour boiling water over the cornmeal and blend into a paste with the vegetable bouillon powder or tamari. Stir until smooth and cook very gently until all the liquid has been absorbed. Cool and drop by the spoonful on to a slightly oiled baking sheet and grill until brown turning once.

Millet (starch)

Once used by the Romans to make porridge, millet is still an important staple in many parts of Africa. It is a bland and highly nutritious grain which contains all of the essential amino acids plus an excellent complement of the B-complex vitamins and minerals.

5 C spring or filtered water
1 C millet
10 ml (2 tsp) vegetable bouillon powder
1 medium onion, chopped finely
5 ml (1 tsp) paprika
30 ml (2 tbsp) chopped parsley, fresh

Boil the water and pour it over the millet in a deep saucepan; then add the vegetable bouillon powder, onion, paprika and half of the parsley. Cook over slow heat for 30–45 minutes until all of the liquid has been absorbed. Sprinkle with the remainder of the parsley and serve. (Cooked millet can be formed into small balls together with grated carrots, finely chopped onions, a little parsley and a little lemon juice and served cold as part of a salad.)

Barley Pilaff (starch)

A delicious baked dish which goes nicely with a living salad. It is made from pot barley, not from pearl barley (too many of the B-complex vitamins and minerals have been removed from pearl barley). Barley is also excellent used in soups.

2 onions, chopped finely
15 ml (1 tbsp) soya or olive oil
1 C pot barley

1½ C spring or filtered water
15 ml (1 tbsp) vegetable bouillon powder
15 ml (1 tbsp) dill
2 cloves of garlic, finely chopped (optional)

Sauté the onions in the oil until translucent, then add the barley, continuing to stir until the grains have become well coated. Remove from the heat and add the remaining ingredients (including the water, boiled in a kettle). Place in a well-oiled oven dish and bake in a moderate oven for half an hour. Check to see if you need to add a little more water. Serve immediately.

Perfect Oatmeal Porridge (starch)

A superb starch meal and an absolute delight to eat in the evening because the high carbohydrate content of porridge has a tendency to increase the brain's uptake of the amino acid tryptophan and therefore to relax you.

1 C porridge oats
3 C spring or filtered water
pinch of sea salt
1 ripe banana
5 ml (1 tsp) cinnamon

Preferably soak the oats for several hours before cooking (you can put them in the pot with the water at lunchtime if the porridge is to be prepared for your evening meal). Heat the porridge and water in a double boiler or place the pan containing the oats and water itself into a large frying pan which contains 2 inches of water. This means that the porridge will cook very slowly and be very smooth. Cook slowly for 15–20 minutes until the mixture has become smooth. If you prefer a thicker mixture you can reduce the amount of water. Remove from stove and pour into a dish with sliced bananas and sprinkle with cinnamon. Serve immediately.

20
On the Go

So there you have it – the principles, the rationale, the guidelines, the recipes and all the rest. Now it is only a question of putting it all into practice and sitting back to enjoy the transformations that are going to take place in your body. But what about special circumstances? For instance, how do you make Raw Energy Food Combining work for you when you have to eat in restaurants, or when you are travelling, or if you want to take your lunch to work or to school with you? It is all a lot easier to cope with than you might imagine.

Lunch is Easy

The business lunch or evening out needn't be a problem. These days more and more restaurants serve decent salads. And, while it is true that most of them are not exactly living delights, they are still a far cry from the traditional limp piece of lettuce with a slice of cucumber, half a tomato and a pale hard-boiled egg.

If you want to eat fish or meat or game then order a dish which is *simply* prepared – not smothered in breadcrumbs (bad starch–protein combination) – such as trout or prawns. If it comes with rice or potatoes ask the waiter if you could please have some vegetables instead and then a mixed or green salad. You can also always order fruit juice or fruit as a starter, provided you leave 20 minutes or more before you start on your next course.

If, like me, you prefer most of the time to stick to vegetable foods, you might order a light green salad to start with and follow that with a plate of whatever the vegetables of the day are. The better the restaurant the more helpful they will be. Most of the time you will be able to order without anybody even suspecting that you are practising conscientious food combining.

If, again like me, you prefer to remain as inconspicuous in your dieting as possible, then it is a good idea to order the same number of courses as the other people you are dining with. You could choose an avocado vinaigrette to start with, for instance, followed by a game main course, some vegetables, and a side salad. Nobody will oblige you to eat pudding these days. I sometimes carry some peppermint tea bags with me as an after-dinner drink while friends are drinking coffee. Then I simply order 'a small pot of tea without the tea please' and pop my bag into it to steep for a couple of minutes when it arrives. By all means enjoy a glass of good wine if you want one.

Friends Can Help

When I was a child my father always accused me of 'stirring my food around my plate' instead of eating it. He is the only person I have ever known who actually noticed that I do this. And it is a great technique to practise when you are in a situation where food combinations have been put on your plate which you do not want to eat (this frequently happens to me at dinner parties). The best way to deal with it is to decide whether you are going to make your meal a protein one or a starch one and then eat only the foods in your selected category, simply moving the rest about on your plate so they look well picked over. When your hostess offers you seconds you can reply with, 'Yes, I would love some more of that delicious rice', or 'Do you think I could have another serving of salad; it's wonderful?' At dinner parties make sure you eat plenty of the side-salads, the vegetables and whatever other neutral foods are available. And don't be afraid to say 'no thank you' when people become persistent with their offers. You can always add, 'It looks lovely but I'm afraid I'm rather full.'

Fly Away

This is easiest of all. Travelling on planes, in the car or on trains is the ideal time to spend a day on fruit or to apple-fast. Not only is it convenient, because you have a ready-made opportunity for not following the standard pattern of three meals a day, it will also help your stamina and your ability to withstand the stress of getting from here to there very well indeed. I never get on an aeroplane for a long flight without a bag of fruit under my arm. Usually it is the most luscious fruit I can find, since I tend rather to spoil myself on the excuse that 'after all, I'm travelling today and so it's rather a special time'. Most airlines these days offer special meals which fit in well with your needs – for instance, fresh fruit salads with yoghurt or cottage cheese, or seafood salads: you need only request them 24 hours before your flight. Once you get used to growing your own sprouts you may even want to carry some of those with you on the go. We often do – especially when we are out hiking (they will grow in plastic bags in a rucksack as well as they do in jars in your kitchen) or when there is a long car journey.

Take It Out

Raw vegetables, fruits or sprouts make excellent foods to put in a lunchbox for school or work. For instance, you can combine any crudités – carrot sticks, celery sticks, broccoli and cauliflower florets, rings or strips of red, yellow and green peppers, mange-tout, diagonal slices of cucumber, courgette, thin slices of Jerusalem artichoke, white radish, kohlrabi, button mushrooms, spring onions, celery hearts, tomatoes, watercress – with a container of rich protein dressing or dip. This makes a delightful lunch. And, provided you keep your fresh vegetables on hand in the refrigerator all cleaned and ready for use as I do, the whole thing will take you no more than five to ten minutes to prepare.

For most people following a Raw Energy Food Combining lifestyle from day to day, being out and about presents little problem. You will probably find after the first few weeks, once you have got the hang of food combining and know pretty well what goes with what, you will not even have to think much about it. After all, if ever things go wrong and you find yourself having eaten a badly combined meal, you can always make the next day an all-raw one or an apple-fast to get yourself back in balance again.

New Life Starts Here

The extraordinary thing about Raw Energy Food Combining is that, once you do get into it, once you have shed your unwanted fat, enhanced your energy levels and are feeling in top form, chances are you are going to want to stick with it. When your body has readjusted itself to its normal weight you can begin to experiment a little. Keep to your food combining but now try eating a few more of your foods cooked. Add more grains to your meals. Try the pulses again, for by now your digestive system will probably have become so much more efficient and so much stronger that you will be able to handle them without difficulty. You will see for yourself how easy it is to take everything you have learned as well as all the positive changes which have happened to you through new ways of eating and exercising and slowly build for yourself a lasting lifestyle for health and good looks. That, after all, is what Raw Energy Food Combining is all about.

BOOK TWO:
JUICE HIGH

To all those who seek the highs
but are devastated by the lows
that usually follow
this little book is dedicated

Contents

1
Lifepower

As soon as you begin to incorporate freshly-extracted, raw vegetable and fruit juices into your lifestyle, something amazing starts happening to you. First you will notice the terrific lift that just one glass of fresh juice can give you, particularly when taken first thing on an empty stomach. Imagine what life might be like if, instead of trying to kick-start yourself with strong coffee in the mornings, you could drink a glass of raw juice and almost immediately feel refreshed, alert and eager to see what another day has in store. This is the liberating effect of the Juice High.

Raw juice is the most perfect fuel for your body. Its high water content means that it is easily assimilated and tends to cleanse and nurture the body while supplying it with a full range of essential nutrients. That's all there is to it. Except, of course, that raw juice also has another property, a mysterious factor X, which scientists have yet to properly understand. Freshly-extracted juices are bursting with *Lifepower* – a natural, raw energy that is miraculous in its beneficial effect on the human body.

The nutritional and recuperative value of raw juice has been well known to doctors and natural health practitioners since the turn of the century, when several of the most eminent pioneers in the field started experimenting with raw foods to improve their own health. The famous **Rohsäft Kur** (raw juice cure) developed by Dr Max Bircher-Benner and Dr Max Gerson nearly ninety years ago is now acknowledged to be the single most potent short-term antidote to fatigue and stress. Until recently

175

it's been the preserve of the privileged few who could afford to go to an exclusive health spa.

Now, with the advent of affordable domestic centrifugal juice extractors, hi-tech nutrition and the salvation of raw juice is within reach. Our raw juice cure – the Juice Blitz (see Chapter 3) – can be undertaken over a weekend in the comfort of your own home. It can be used as a quick-fix detox programme, or as the first step towards changing your life.

Raw Energy Rush

Energy is the essence of life, the force that makes everything feasible and achievable. In the body, energy is produced by billions of tiny powerhouses – or cells – and for our bodies to function at peak efficiency, we must provide the optimum conditions for each cell to do its work. In order to be fit and healthy and to live a long and active life, we need plenty of fresh air and the vital nourishment that comes from eating whole foods.

Only in comparatively recent times has mankind come to realise that the condition of the human body is inextricably bound up with the quality of the food we ingest and the air we breathe. Over the past hundred years, since the Industrial Revolution, the quality of both our food and air and consequently our ability to be healthy has declined dramatically. Because we now live in an environment that is increasingly toxic, we need the most effective form of nutrition in order to combat its degenerative effects and to revitalise our bodies.

Not only do our bodies need the full range of essential nutrients to be healthy, but they need them to be available in the form in which they can most readily be utilised. That means *in the raw*. Raw fruits and vegetables contain the most valuable array of vitamins, minerals and amino acids, but they also have a uniquely healthful quality which science has yet to decode. Since scientists cannot formulate into pills nutrients they haven't yet identified, the biggest synthetic vitamin pill you can buy can never compensate for a lack of the natural goodness that is only contained within raw fruits and vegetables.

The simple reason why raw juices are so beneficial is because they deliver, straight into your system, the most complete range of nutrients in their most vital form, suspended in water from an organic source and brimming with enzymes. Enzymes are the intangible living elements which act as the catalyst for innumerable chemical reactions within the body, promoting efficient assimilation and enabling the metabolic processes that support high levels of energy and promote good health.

Good health should not be defined as the absence of disease, but as a vital, dynamic condition in which we feel positively charged and fully able to take whatever life has to throw at us. This is the property we call Raw Energy and the most immediate way to experience its Lifepower is by drinking raw juice.

Re: Juice

Replenishment is the immutable law of life. If we fail to replace the water in our bodies that is lost through perspiration, we become dehydrated and soon start to wilt. The soft drinks industry is a big and rapidly growing business that churns out billions of bucks' worth of propaganda to persuade us that cans of carbonated syrup will satisfy our thirst and enhance our energy. There's even a breed of so-called 'sports drinks' which are claimed not only to replace bodily fluids, but also to reinvigorate tired muscles. Actually, the last thing most of these synthetic products can offer your body is proper refreshment and, while they may give you a sugar shock or a caffeine jolt, as a source of prolonged energy they are worthless.

In fact, the kind of water your body craves and depends upon to function at peak efficiency does not come out of a tap, or from a bottle, but is only found in fresh fruits and vegetables. Your body can't use the water in fizzy drinks, or beer, and so those fluids pass quickly through to the bladder. The water extracted from raw fruit and vegetables, however, has a unique organic quality and is readily absorbed by the body. Because it is so rich in essential micro-nutrients, raw juice effectively replenishes lost energy. In fact, raw juice is the most profoundly refreshing fluid you can drink.

Fatal Fizz

People working in the soul-sapping environment of, say, a modern office building will reach for coffee and fizzy drinks in the middle of the afternoon in the hope that it will give them enough mental energy to make it through to the end of another hectic day. Then they experience a corresponding energy slump on the way home, arriving irritable and exhausted and good for nothing but going early to bed. The end result of living like this is a kind of chronic fatigue that often manifests itself as indifferent, fatalistic lethargy.

So-called 'soft drinks' bring nutritionally empty calories into your body which you can ill afford. A twelve ounce can of cola contains seven teaspoons (40 g) of sugar and is full of chemicals that pollute your body, including phosphoric acid – the chemical used to etch glass – which impedes the function of the kidneys and leaches calcium from bones, teeth and hair. As for the 'diet' varieties, quite apart from the proven fact that drinking them will do absolutely nothing to help you lose weight, they are an even more noxious cocktail of artificial chemicals. Stay away from them.

But the main reason you will want to abandon soft drinks and make raw juice your preferred beverage is because it tastes fantastic. If you've tried bottled carrot juice and didn't like it, don't be put off from tasting the real thing. Freshly-extracted carrot juice is sweet, creamy and delicious. Mix it with apple juice and you have a whole drink that is perfectly balanced for your nutritional needs, but also tastes so good that we have never come across anyone who doesn't like it.

Pure Fuel

All our energy is ultimately derived from the food we eat and without proper digestion there can be no such thing as good nutrition. Food passes through the body, from the oesophagus via the stomach and gastro-intestinal tract, where it is broken down and nutrients are assimilated into the body. Although it's true that we are what we eat, it's more accurate to say that we are what we assimilate. By extracting the juices of fruits and vegetables, removing their fibre, we can provide the body with an excellent source of nutrition that is virtually pre-digested, so that it is assimilated with minimum effort.

No less important than efficient assimilation is the prompt elimination of food wastes that will otherwise accumulate in the colon and decay, breeding putrefactive bacteria that release toxins which get into the bloodstream, spreading all sorts of sickness throughout the body. The residues of digested food pass from the small intestine into the colon in liquid form and are moved along by the action of peristalsis, to be eliminated from the bowels. The fibres in raw foods assist this process, acting as a kind of intestinal broom, but when food is denatured by processing, the action is more like a filthy mop that leaves a trail of slime coating the intestinal walls and making the colon sluggish and slow.

There is nothing in raw juice that your body cannot use and, therefore, nothing that it need work to expel. Instead, the body can concentrate on getting rid of old waste and the action of raw juice will encourage that by irrigating the intestine and causing a chain reaction in the colon that can have explosive results! This laxative effect, which is particularly pronounced with fruit juices, is highly beneficial because it helps the body to detoxify itself, providing the ideal environment for biological regeneration.

Rejuvenation

As you become accustomed to juicing, and to the effect of raw juice on your bowel movements, you may well shed excess weight. As your colon cleanses itself and your metabolism becomes more efficient, and so long as you are not continually clogging your system with junk foods, the body will revert to its natural weight. You start to feel fitter and younger than you have in years and you get used to old friends telling you how well you look. What's more, when you see yourself in the mirror, you even *look* younger; your complexion seems smoother and wrinkles recede. This is no illusion. The Lifepower of freshly-extracted juices has the potential to rejuvenate your body in a way that quite literally makes you younger.

What makes us old is not merely the passing years but environmental poisons, inadequate food and mental stress. These factors conspire to cause an acidic chemical imbalance within the body that is redressed by raw juice, which tends to be alkaline. One of the most significant factors in premature ageing is the effect of free radical particles in atmospheric pollution, biochemical bully boys that vandalise our bodies at a cellular level. The best way to combat them is with a regular intake of raw juice.

Smog Off

The infernal internal combustion engine has proved to be the most destructive invention of the twentieth century and it's going to be difficult to explain to future generations why we allowed their air to be poisoned by exhaust fumes and condemned them to grow up with a range of respiratory illnesses caused by pollution. Just breathe in by the side of the road and savour that acrid cocktail of sulphur dioxide and carbon monoxide, liberally laced with benzene and hydrocarbons.

Your body is a biochemical battleground in which the baddies are the free radicals that are particularly prevalent in car exhaust fumes. Scientifically, free radicals are molecules with an unpaired electron, which makes them highly reactive and inclined to stabilise themselves by attracting another electron from any other molecule, particularly the lipids in cell membranes. These are the fundamental building blocks of our bodily tissues. By knocking out a few of these blocks in a process called 'lipid peroxidation', free radicals can bring the whole lot tumbling down by causing an ever-amplifying series of chain reactions that leads to the destruction of tissues. That's how smoking and breathing heavily-polluted air corrodes our vitality, causes cancer and makes us old before our time.

Still, what can you do? Walking around in a hi-tech gas mask is hardly practicable, so you'd better ensure you get yourself a plentiful supply of the fresh vitamins that can prevent or retard free radical damage. You need plenty of A, C and E, the so-called anti-oxidant vitamins, as well as other recently-discovered plant-based anti-oxidant compounds that are found only in fresh fruit and vegetables, to protect yourself against the degenerative effects of pollution. The best way to ensure an adequate supply is . . . to drink plenty of freshly-extracted raw juice.

Food Glut

A potentially catastrophic revolution has taken place in our eating habits over the past century. Commercial considerations, rather than concern for human health, have been allowed to dictate the way in which our food is produced, processed and distributed. Crops are grown in chemically-fertilised soils, doused with pesticides and then made into products which are packaged to be shipped over long distances and stored for extended periods. All these complicated modern practices conspire to destroy the wholesome quality of the foodstuffs we can most easily afford to buy from the local supermarket.

The convenience foods that dominate the diets of most of us privileged to be living in the affluent, developed world have had their nutritional integrity destroyed. Their natural goodness has been systematically stripped from them and replaced with a range of artificial additives to enhance their taste and mouthfeel and to prolong their shelf life as far as possible. Refined foods are loaded with excessive amounts of fats and sugars, but offer the body practically nothing in terms of nutrition, failing adequately to satisfy our appetite for real food and tempting us to overeat, compulsively.

Fat Chances

Widespread obesity is a relatively new phenomenon, but one which is now a contributing factor in a range of chronic degenerative diseases that have become the biggest killers of modern times: cardiovascular conditions and cancer. While it is possible to subsist on a diet of microwavable ready meals, it's impossible to thrive. Despite the miracles of medical science, statistics demonstrate that the population as a whole is not getting healthier.

A poor diet undermines good health and leaves you in

poor shape to cope with the stresses and strains of modern life but, much worse, it's bad for the soul. The physiological effect of a high-gunk diet – that's one that tends to clog your system with rubbish that's nutritionally worthless and hard to digest – is to slow you down, making you feel heavy. Psychologically, that can only make you depressed.

Stop Wilting

Before World War II all crops were grown without the use of chemicals, which is to say organically. The organic matter in healthy soil creates fertility and promotes the growth of strong, healthy plants. Artificial chemicals interfere with that vital process, stripping the soil of its natural goodness and depriving the plants grown in it of essential minerals and other micro-substances. Destroy the soil's organic matter through chemical farming, and slowly, but inexorably, the health of people and animals that live on the foods grown in it will be undermined and their resistance to disease will be compromised.

The body has an amazing ability to compensate for missing nutrients, but after years of eating nutritionally depleted foods, widespread deficiencies are becoming apparent and all sorts of metabolic distortions follow. Being fat is the most obvious one, but perhaps the most insidious effect of the modern diet is the imbalance of sodium and potassium in many people's bodies.

Sodium and potassium are nutritional antagonists that act synergistically in the body to regulate the osmotic pressure on the walls of each cell. When properly balanced, these two minerals also transmit electrochemical impulses throughout the body, keeping the whole organism vibrant. Too much sodium or too little potassium and the organism starts to wilt, causing the kind of chronic fatigue that has you reaching for coffee and chocolate biscuits in the middle of the afternoon just to keep going.

That is what's happening to masses of people nowadays who have too much salt in their diet, promoting acidity in the body and undermining its resilience. What they need is potassium and the best way to get it – you've guessed it – is by drinking raw juice.

Get Smart

There's nothing controversial in the suggestion that eating fresh fruit and vegetables will significantly reduce your chances of dying prematurely from heart disease or cancer. The World Health Organisation recommends that we eat at least half a kilo of fresh fruit and vegetables every day. When the Europe Against Cancer campaign launched its 'Five-A-Day' initiative, aimed at encouraging the daily intake of at least five hundred-gramme portions of fruit and vegetables, they pointed out that Britain falls far short of the target, with the lowest fruit and vegetable consumption – and the highest incidence of heart disease – in Europe.

It's not just adults who require the raw energy of fresh foods to thrive. Unborn babies are particularly vulnerable: thousands have been born with spina bifida because their mothers were deficient in folic acid during the first six weeks of pregnancy, perhaps before many of them even realised they were pregnant. Folic acid is a soluble vitamin, a member of the B complex, which assists the formation of DNA. It's abundant in green vegetables like broccoli, but is easily destroyed by cooking.

Many children refuse to eat enough fresh vegetables because they say they don't like the taste. Sadly, many kids these days are addicted to sugar and so used to sloppy convenience foods that they can't be bothered to chew whole food properly. But fresh juices are easy to drink and it's no problem to persuade children to take them, since they taste delicious.

Get Juicing

Never forget that the body and mind are not separate entities, but are completely interdependent. The foods we consume dictate not only our physical well-being, but our moods and ability to think clearly. People who are in control of their health are in control of their destiny, able to work harder and more effectively to fulfil their dreams.

Once you start to incorporate freshly-extracted raw fruits and vegetable juices into your diet you will begin to arrest the build-up of toxins in your body. As you continue to take raw juices on a regular basis, the deadly degenerative effects of a junk diet will be reversed. This process of detoxification may be gradual or it may be quite dramatic, depending on the enthusiasm with which you take to raw juice, but its effects are always remarkable.

Raw juice will help you to build the stamina to cope with the debilitating stresses of modern life, but it can also transform the way you see the world around you. As your body re-balances itself, you'll find that your moods stabilise, too. Trivialities cease to upset you and you are able to keep things in perspective. Detoxifying the system and flushing your colon with raw juice actually helps you to think more clearly and rationally, to concentrate for longer and maintain a more optimistic frame of mind. This is the state we call Juice High and, unlike the high you get from coffee, or drugs, it is perfectly possible to stay high on raw juice all of the time.

Drinking raw juice is not like doing drugs. Drug users often say they are seeking enlightenment, to 'expand their minds', but by artificially altering their perceptions with chemicals they may be doing themselves damage. Whether or not drugs do long-term harm, their effects are temporary and usually followed by a 'crash' when the drug wears off. (Drinking raw juice, by the way, is the best possible thing you can do to recover from the after-effects of drug abuse or excessive drinking.) People take drugs to get 'out of it' and 'off their heads' but raw juice will have the opposite effect, making you feel more 'normal', better 'centred', and properly 'connected'.

Any raw juice is better than none at all, but if you use your juice well, and take it on a daily basis, you might just come to realise that, since you started juicing, not only has your health perked up, you feel positively happy.

2
Get Juiced

Harmony is the underlying principle of life. All illnesses can be regarded as a manifestation of disharmony within the human body.

If all the metabolic processes that animate your body and enable you to live a fully active and healthy life are to work properly, the internal environment of the body requires perfect harmony. Breathing polluted air and eating processed foods replete with sugar, junk fats and refined carbohydrates (not to mention bad habits like drinking and smoking) conspire to create excess acidity and create a chemical imbalance within the body. All raw juices have a strongly alkalinising effect, tipping the pH balance back to normal, helping to restore harmony and enabling the body to cleanse and heal itself.

Juice It

There are three clearly defined stages in the body's utilisation of food: appropriation (eating and digestion); assimilation (taking in nutrients) and elimination (expelling waste products). While all these activities are always taking place to some extent, the function of each is heightened at different times during the course of a day. If you've ever slumped on the sofa after a big meal, unable to move, you'll know how much energy the process of breaking down food in the stomach requires. If you really stuff yourself, your body is forced to close down some of your other physiological functions while it gets to grips with digesting.

Because it requires so much energy, the body prefers

to do most of the hard work of assimilation at night, while you sleep. By the time you wake up in the morning, you will have moved into the elimination cycle. This is not a matter of having a single bowel movement before breakfast, but a deep and thorough cleansing at cellular level, with wastes being expelled via all the organs of elimination, including the skin and lungs as well as the bowels and urinary tract. The elimination cycle lasts throughout the morning and that is the best time to take raw juices, particularly those freshly extracted from fruit.

Fruit juices are great for getting you moving in the mornings. All fruit contains fructose, the natural sugar that your body can use for fuel, and is usually around 90 per cent water, promoting prompt elimination. When perfectly ripe, fruit also contains its own digestive enzymes and is therefore virtually pre-digested – it passes rapidly through the stomach and into the intestines. Of course, fruit juices can cause a rapid rise in blood sugar, so diabetics and people who are prone to yeast infections should be careful how they use them, but most people will find the effect of a glass of raw fruit juice for breakfast quite invigorating. Drink a glass of freshly extracted watermelon, or pineapple, or pink grapefruit juice on an empty stomach and within fifteen minutes you'll be wide awake and ready to rock.

It is always best to take fruits or their juices on an empty stomach, since they cannot be so effective if their passage through the stomach is impeded by undigested food. In fact, resolving to consume nothing but raw juices and fruit from the moment you get up until lunchtime could well be the healthiest lifestyle decision you ever make. As the day progresses, incorporate more and more vegetables into your juices and switch their emphasis from sweet to savoury.

The Juice Kitchen

Undoubtedly the most useful tool in the juice kitchen is a vegetable peeler. Not a blunt old potato peeler, but a speed peeler with a pivoting head which can be bought from any catering supply shop if you can't find one in the local hardware store. Not all vegetables should be peeled, however, as their nutrients tend to be concentrated in the skin. Organic carrots, beetroots and apples are great juiced whole. Buy a scrubbing brush such as a nail brush to scrub the dirt off root vegetables. The brush will also be useful for scrubbing the strainer basket of your juicer.

Second, you need a sharp knife and a cutting board. If your chosen juicer has a spout rather than an integral jug, find some glasses that fit snugly under the spout, but buy an accurate measuring jug as well and use it to formulate your own recipes. Juicing directly into the glass saves on washing up, but it's useful to have a swizzle stick – a chop-stick will do – or a thin wooden spoon to stir your juices before serving.

Third, of course, you need a juicer – and it really does have to be more sophisticated than the traditional hand-held push-down-and-turn conical object at the back of your kitchen cupboard.

Buying a Juicer

Centrifugal juice extractors contain a basket, usually made from stainless steel, with sharp shredding blades at the bottom and a fine mesh screen at the sides. When you push fruit and vegetables through the rotating blades, the pulp is spun off into a receptacle at the back of the machine and the juice strained out through a spout, or into an integral jug. A juicer with a spout is better than one with a jug because then you can juice directly into a glass and there's less to wash up.

As with any domestic appliance, look for the most

robust model you can get for your money. This means the one with the strongest motor and the strongest locking mechanism. Beware of two-speed juicers and those models with a hopper that simply clicks into place without your having to clamp it down. These rinky-dink features just give you more to go wrong.

One other thing to check before buying your juicer is the size of the hole you are supposed to put the produce through. Some are really too small and it's a drag to have to slice even the skinniest carrot lengthways.

Russell once took a burned-out juicer back to the shop when it was less than a year old and the salesman asked how much he had used it. Actually, he'd used it every day, but what was it designed for? Don't be afraid to demand a demonstration of the model you intend to buy, listen to the whine the motor makes and ask yourself if it sounds as if it can stand up to the job.

For details of other equipment, see Resources, pages 432–3.

Next to Godliness

Cleanliness is important with regard to the proper maintenance of your juicer, which will quickly become stained unless you take proper care of it. The strong natural pigments of the raw foods you'll be juicing will inevitably stain the plastic parts of your juicer, so that you will have to soak them regularly in a bleach solution to keep your machine pristine. More importantly, you must thoroughly scour your juicer every time you use it with plenty of hot water, ensuring that the steel basket that does the work of shredding is absolutely clean and that there are no bits of vegetable matter caught in the fine mesh of the sieve.

It's always easier to clean your juicer straight after you've used it than it will be the next time you want to use it. We find that it's good practice to clean the juicer before drinking the juice we've just made. That way, we're so eager to get the chore over with that the work takes only a minute.

Get Freshness

Freshness is the first principle of good juicing. When buying fresh produce, don't let yourself be palmed off with overripe fruit that's started to 'turn', or soft and sad-looking vegetables with limp leaves. Choose only the most perfectly ripe fruits and vegetables and don't buy more than you can use over a couple of days. You will be getting through a lot of produce, but don't be tempted to buy in bulk unless you're sure you're going to use it up. While it's often not necessary to peel the produce you'll be juicing, it *is* essential to wash it thoroughly, using a scrubbing brush if necessary, under cold running water.

Freshly-extracted juices must be drunk as soon as they are made, before their Raw Energy expires. The nutrients in raw juice are highly volatile and will begin to deteriorate as soon as they are in contact with fresh air, so that its essential vitality is quickly lost. If you want to demonstrate this for yourself, leave a glass of raw juice to stand for just a few minutes and you'll see how quickly it separates into a clear liquid (water) with a scummy head on top. A lot less inviting than the vividly coloured fluid you started with. Stir the scum back into the liquid before drinking it and you'll notice a marked deterioration in the taste.

It's best not to try storing raw juices, but they can be kept in the fridge for a couple of hours, with a lid on the container. When going on a journey, or forced to spend the day in the alien environment of an office, we do find it beneficial to take along a flask of raw juice to keep us going. Use a large, wide-necked, insulated flask and insert a couple of ice cubes before pouring in your freshly-extracted juice. That way the juice will keep for half a day or longer without losing too much of its wholesomeness. This is definitely a superior refreshment to canned soft drinks.

The Basics

So far, we've talked of fresh fruits and vegetables in more or less the same breath, but before you begin juicing it's important to understand that the two types of juice act within the body in quite different ways. Basically, *fruit* is liquid brain fuel that is particularly useful for detoxifying your body and clearing your mind, while *vegetables* provide the nutritional blocks for rebuilding the metabolic machinery of your body.

Some juice enthusiasts will warn you not to combine fruit and vegetable juices in the same glass, lest they give you wind and cause embarrassing flatulence. In fact this doesn't always happen. The two types of juice can be combined satisfactorily, but in general they don't tend to taste so good together. The exceptions are carrot and apple, which can be mixed with anything.

Carrot is King

During the World War II, propagandists covered up the invention of radar by trying to persuade the enemy that allied fighter pilots were eating so many carrots that they could see in the dark! This hyperbole does, however, contain a grain of truth. Carrots have been repeatedly shown to nourish the optic nerve and significantly improve eyesight in general and night vision in particular. This is but one of the healing properties of the humble carrot, which is the richest source of beta-carotene, the vegetable pigment that gives carrots their glorious orange colour and which the body converts into the cancer-fighting antioxidant, vitamin A.

Carrots also contain vitamins C and E, as well as B, D, G and K and the minerals calcium, sodium, potassium, iron and phosphorus. Carrot juice is composed of a combination of elements which nourish the entire system, helping the body to normalize its weight and restore its chemical balance. CJ is incredibly good for you, but recent reports have suggested that eating carrots could be harmful because they contain poisonous pesticide residues.

Not long ago the UK Pesticides Safety Directorate issued a warning after scientists found carrot pesticide residues 25 times higher than they had expected and, in some cases, three times higher than the accepted safety level. The Food Minister was moved to advise the public to remove the tops and peel all carrots, as if that would make them safe. Sadly, the systemic organophosphates concerned don't stop at the skin, they penetrate the whole vegetable. Naturally, therefore, it is always preferable to use organic produce wherever possible.

When it comes to juicing, the carrot is king. It is the most versatile vegetable, with the sweetest juice. If you've only ever tried bottled carrot juice, and didn't like it, don't be put off from trying freshly-extracted CJ, which tastes sublime.

The carotene content of carrots varies considerably and is reflected in the colour. Carrots bought from the supermarket are sometimes almost fluorescent, while organic carrots are a much deeper shade of orange, indicating a much higher concentration of carotene. When buying carrots, choose those with the darkest colour. Although size doesn't really matter, where the recipes in this book refer to a carrot or a number of carrots, as a guide these should be around 15cm (6in) in length.

Whichever variety you use, you'll need about a pound, or half a kilo, of carrots to make 280ml or 10 fl.oz juice.

As a rule of thumb, we reckon that half a dozen medium carrots will yield about half a pint of juice. Scrub them under cold running water and remove the tops and tails, but it is not necessary to peel carrots before putting them through the juicer.

Have a Go

Carrot and apple – don't call it Crapple – is the most basic juice cocktail and it tastes so good that, in our experience, nobody has ever turned their nose up at it! Use the *whole* apple except for the woody stem. Apple seeds contain important nourishment too. Start by combining equal parts of the two juices and experiment until you find the proportions that suit you – half and half perhaps, or one part apple to two parts carrot.

Apples are Ace!

If an apple a day keeps the doctor away, a glass or two of freshly-extracted apple juice will keep you regular, boost your immunity to colds, and keep your hair and nails looking lustrous. Apples are full of the soluble dietary fibre, pectin, which makes the juice cloudy, gives it a delightfully creamy texture and acts in the body to clean out toxins and relieve constipation. Apples are also rich in beta-carotene and vitamin C, as well as several B-complex vitamins including B6, and the mineral potassium.

Just as the carrot is the most versatile vegetable when it comes to juicing, apples are the most useful fruit. Apple juice can happily be mixed with any vegetable juice. As such, it is particularly useful in enabling those who are new to juicing slowly to acclimatize themselves to the earthy, wild, raw taste of some freshly extracted juices. Start off by incorporating a lot of apple and gradually reduce the proportion as you become accustomed to the taste and texture of raw juice.

You may be familiar with the taste of juice pressed from various varieties of apple, but you might be surprised by how sweetly smooth and creamy freshly-extracted apple juice is. There are dozens of apple varieties, each with its own distinct flavour, and it's fun to try each one as it appears. In general, you'll find that the greener the apple, the sharper its juice. Golden Delicious are popular, but we find Cox's ideal.

There's no need to peel apples (in fact it's better if you don't) but do wash them thoroughly. Remove the stalk, but not the core. Simply chop them in half and put them through the juicer.

Apples and pears are closely related, but pear trees are less hardy and the fruit more perishable. Pear juice is thick, mild and versatile. It mixes well with other juices, and can be a useful substitute for apple in many recipes. Pears should be washed and the stem removed, then cut to fit your juicer. Mix the juice of two pears with the juice of two apples and drink it down promptly, since this combination oxidizes quickly.

Bring on the Berries

Berries are intensely-flavoured vitamin bombs that tend to be high in potassium and contain a remarkable range of other trace elements. Berries have been shown to be particularly good for fighting 'flu and preventing cancer. Strawberries, raspberries, blackberries . . . in fact any berry works well when blended with apple juice, or apple and pear. Juice two apples, one pear and as many berries as you like, or can fit into the glass.

Berries are replete with something called *ellegic acid* – a natural plant *phenol* which is believed to be a powerful anti-cancer/anti-ageing compound. Researchers working with it believe that ellegic acid probably has protective properties because it is taken up by receptor sites that are also used by chemically-induced carcinogens. Animal experiments have demonstrated just how powerful a protective effect ellegic-acid-containing foods have when researchers fed mice on them and then deliberately applied a nasty cancer-causing polycyclic aromatic hydrocarbon (PAH) to the skin for several weeks. The berry-eaters had 45 per cent fewer tumours than the control group and the latency period before they appeared was stretched from six to ten weeks. Berries are also high in potassium and rich in iron. Some, like blackcurrants and redcurrants also contain GLA (a health-giving fatty acid), others like cranberries are great for clearing urinary and bladder infections.

Taking the Pith

When juicing citrus fruit, remove the peel but leave as much of the white pith as you like to get the full benefit of the bioflavonoids contained within it, which help the body to absorb vitamin C. Bioflavonoids are powerful plant-based anti-oxidants. They also have an ability to strengthen the capillaries in the body which carry nutrients to the cells via the bloodstream. This means better circulation and smoother, more beautiful skin. The juice of citrus fruits squeezed on a conventional cone juicer often has bits of pith floating in it, which have an unpleasant feel in the mouth. It tends to taste sharp and to cause acidity within the body. Juice that's made using a centrifugal extractor, however, is a whole food in which the citric acid is neutralized by the bioflavonoids, providing the body with a well-balanced drink that can be readily assimilated. It's also absolutely delicious and has a wonderful, creamy texture; it has a sweetness quite unlike squeezed juice.

Citrus juices are jam-packed with fruit sugar and bursting with vitamin C, helping to crank up the immune system and providing instant energy. We find a big glass of frothy pink grapefruit juice just the thing to get us started on a miserable, wet winter morning.

The Whole Juice

The seeds in fruits such as apples and oranges are enormously rich in nutrients. The orange seed has nine times more calcium, seven times more magnesium, and more potassium than an equal amount of orange juice. Apple seeds have five times more potassium than extracted apple juice. Other seeds – those from the rose family such as cherries, peaches, plums, apricots and apples – contain a very small amount of a chemical called amygdalin which is believed to release minute quantities of cyanide. This is not anything that one should be overly concerned about since you would have to consume 50–100 apricot stones to take in a harmful dose. However, we do not suggest you put apricot or cherry stones into the juicer, as they will only blunt the blades.

Go with the Flow

Raw juices are incredibly rich in nutrients and they have a powerful effect on our health, but it would be quite wrong to describe them as 'concentrated'. As you get into juicing and begin talking to friends about it, you will almost inevitably come across someone who'll try to warn you that too much of a good thing can be bad for you. They might cite the dimly-remembered case of some health fanatic who killed himself with carrot juice. That did actually happen, but the person involved was not only drinking several *gallons* of fresh CJ per day, he was also guzzling toxic doses of vitamin A tablets over months and years to the point where his liver gave up on him. Obviously, he was overdoing it.

When raw juices were first discussed in medical and

scientific arenas, it was suggested that they should only be taken in tiny doses, but this was undoubtedly because there wasn't a machine on the market that could easily extract juice in any quantity. Imagine what price you'd put on a glass of carrot juice if you had to grate the vegetable and somehow force it through a super-fine strainer by hand. Now that we have handy centrifugal machines, the recommendation is that you must consume at least a pint of raw juice every day to begin to feel the beneficial effects.

It's true that some juices are very potent and should only be taken in small quantities. However, it will be immediately apparent to you which these juices are because they also have an intensely powerful taste and are too strong to drink straight. Juices are supposed to taste pleasant! The juices of beetroot and broccoli and all leafy, dark green vegetables must be diluted by at least four times the quantity of much milder juices, like carrot and apple, to be palatable.

When you first start juicing, you may well experience some slight discomfort as your body purges itself of toxins and starts to sort itself out, but this is transitory and only to be expected. It's a good idea to start slowly, with no more than a couple of glasses of juice each day. It is virtually impossible to overdose on raw juice – so long, that is, as you don't try to force unnatural quantities of the stuff down yourself. Drink only as much raw juice as feels comfortable. The juices are so delicious you may be tempted to gulp them down. Don't. It is important to drink your juices slowly, sipping them so that all their goodness is absorbed, nothing is wasted and they mix well with salivary enzymes.

The Spice of Life

As you get into juicing and become accustomed to the staple combinations, you will soon lose any inhibitions you may have nurtured about tasting more pungent and increasingly earthy juices. It's important that you do. Carrot & Apple, or Carrot & Orange juices are all very well, in fact they're terrific. But to derive the maximum benefit from your juicer, it's vital that you consume as broad a variety of fruits and vegetables as possible. Leafy green vegetables are particularly important for good health, as we'll see in Chapter Seven, but they can taste foul at first. The trick is to gradually incorporate more green – more cabbage, spinach, dandelion, etc – into your juices as you become accustomed to the taste.

Raw juices can be spiced up with the addition of root ginger, or fresh garlic, but easy does it. Both have strong flavours, which can be overpowering, and garlic in particular can have an overwhelming effect. Don't use more than one clove per glass of juice and wash the juicer out thoroughly immediately after using garlic, for it is likely to become contaminated and to continue flavouring your juices for days to come. Ginger need not be peeled, just cut into cubes of about a centimetre.

However you choose to get into juicing, the important thing is simply to get started and see where it takes you. Juice-making is a highly creative sport. There is always some delicious new combination just waiting to be discovered.

3
Juice Blitz

'Detox' has become a buzz-word of the late 20th and early 21st centuries, but it is not a recent fad. For thousands of years, detoxification rituals have been used by mystics and shamen in order to retain a state of heightened spirituality. Ritual fasting, with the conviction that abstinence brings us closer to God, is a feature of many religions. On a secular level, many Westerners periodically spend time at health farms in order to give their battered bodies a break from rich food, poor air and the stresses and strains of modern life.

Detoxification is the process of eliminating stored wastes from the body and is the first step in curing addiction. If you are determined to give up cigarettes, for example, the Juice Blitz will help you. By consuming nothing but raw juice and spring water for 36 hours, not only will you remove the temptation to smoke after meals or over a drink, but you will facilitate the process of elimination and help to flush the nicotine out of your body. In fact, the Juice Blitz can be a useful tool in the withdrawal stage of treatment for any form of substance abuse. Then, of course, the addict has to alter the behavioural patterns that reinforce his or her addiction.

Juice High

If you have never, ever, over-indulged in any processed or chemically-treated or preserved food, if you've never smoked a cigarette, done drugs or got drunk, then you probably don't need to detox your body. But how many of us have led that kind of blameless and boring life?

Bearing in mind all the junk you've put into your body over the years, you'll realize that you can't get rid of it all overnight. Like housework, the Juice Blitz takes a little effort, but the end result more than makes it all worthwhile. It's not easy to change the eating habits of a lifetime, but the Juice Blitz will enable you to make a fresh start.

Juice Freedom

Remember that there is nothing in raw juice that your body can't use. By going for 36 hours without consuming anything but raw juice, you will be giving your body a break and relieving it of the hard work of digestion. Left to its own devices, the body will automatically initiate a wholesale house-cleaning. A small minority of people find this process uncomfortable. If you experience any of the reactions described in the 'Trouble Shooting' table (see pages 215–16), take it as an indication that this cleansing process is well under way and that your body is purging itself. And be glad for that.

You may be pleasantly surprised by the effect that blitzing your body has on your mind. Many people experience an amazing mind lift almost as soon as they stop clogging their bodies with junk and start flushing their system. Considering the synergistic relationship of the body and mind, it should be obvious that lightening the body's workload will free the mind to roam fresh horizons.

Fasting on raw juices is probably the most potent short-term antidote to stress. What's more, we find that if we have a lot of work to do that requires our full concentration over long periods, it's also a great way to meet deadlines! Whenever we feel run-down and jaded, or in need of a clearer head, the Juice Blitz can not only reinvigorate our bodies, but also clear mental blockages, and help us to get a better perspective on difficult problems or vexatious situations. Sometimes, we find ourselves living on nothing but raw juice for a day or two at a stretch just because it feels so good.

Crash Detox

The Juice Blitz is a crash course designed to introduce novices to the state of being Juice High. It can be performed at home over the weekend since this will probably give you a chance for more rest. From, say, Friday night to Sunday lunchtime, all you will be putting into your body is freshly-extracted raw juice. If this sounds arduous, then be reassured that you won't go hungry. Although it doesn't sit heavily in your stomach, raw juice completely satisfies the appetite. Most people find themselves perfectly happy with four to six glasses over the course of the day. However, you can drink more than that so long as you don't overdo it. Have spring water too, if you like. Let your body be the judge of how much you need.

The eight juice recipes given below demonstrate some of the classic juice combinations that you might use after, as well as during, your Juice Blitz. They promote effective elimination and provide all the raw energy your body needs for the valuable work of deep cleansing. They are listed in the order that they should be consumed during the day, with the fruit juices to be drunk in the morning and the more savoury, earthier vegetable cocktails to be taken as the day wears on. You're not required to make use of all these recipes, or even to stick to them. The recipes are highly adaptable (for more variations see Recipes, p.289) and the possible combinations of raw juice are infinite, so feel free to improvise. But don't abandon the principle of drinking fruit juices *before* vegetable juices. Here is what the Blitz regime looks like:

THE NIGHT BEFORE

Start your Juice Blitz by going to bed a little hungry the night before. For dinner, drink a glass of the More Raw NRG cocktail or Potassium Punch (see pages 209 and 210). These are ideal, because their exceptional potassium content will counteract the acidity in your body and set up the optimum conditions for your body to do its work. Unless diluted with spring water, the root vegetable drinks may seem a little heavy for beginners to handle at this early stage in the game.

JUICE BLITZ DAY

Start the next morning with a melon or citrus juice and continue with fruit juices until midday. For lunch, try one of the more potent vegetable cocktails, like the Beet Treat (see page 210), which is a great source of sustained energy to carry you through the day. Throughout the afternoon and early evening, stick to vegetable juices in which apple is the only fruit ingredient. We find the More Raw NRG cocktail (see page 209) to be the most useful while detoxing, adding dark green leaves of spinach or watercress or even dandelion to increase its vitality.

Over the course of the first day of a juice fast, you may experience the odd sensation that is not entirely pleasurable. You might find yourself suddenly irritable, or tired, or you could even develop a mild headache. The best antidote to any of these symptoms is to lie down in a darkened room and take a nap. If you have been able to give over your weekend to the Juice Blitz, rest as much as possible and let your body do its work in peace. In any case, rest as much as possible. Don't attempt any strenuous exercise while you are blitzing, but a gentle stroll in fresh air is always a good idea.

BLITZ NIGHT & MORNING AFTER

On Blitz night avoid consuming anything except water after 8 o'clock. You might like to take a long, languorous bath. If you can find a friend to share it with and scrub your back, so much the better. Perhaps your friend can be persuaded to give you a massage as well. The best thing to do on Saturday night while you're blitzing is to go to bed early and get a good night's sleep. If you're not sleepy, go to bed anyway. If you're going to bed alone, take a juicy novel or a lurid video to keep yourself entertained.

The morning after, start the day once again with fruit juice. After a good night's rest, you are likely to be feeling full of the joys of life. Even if your night was not particularly restful and you found yourself waking at dawn in a pool of sweat, you will probably feel sharper, mentally. If you customarily do a crossword in the Sunday papers, we bet you'll find that you finish it faster than usual. You may also find sudden surges of energy, accompanied by some mental agitation. These are both symptoms that your metabolism has been cranked into high gear and the best antidote is a brisk walk in fresh air.

RAW ENERGY LUNCH

As you approach lunchtime on the second day and the end of your Juice Blitz, you may be faced with the predicament of having to sit down to a large, traditional meal or risk offending your mum, or the person who cooked it. You might even be looking forward to stuffing yourself. Don't. Your first meal should be composed of at least 75 per cent raw foods. That means plenty of salad . . .

Ease yourself back into the routine of normal meals by

eating smaller portions and by taking care to chew every mouthful thoroughly. That way you will be better able to appreciate the taste of your food and it will be digested more quickly.

THE REST OF YOUR LIFE

Should you wish to carry on blitzing and to continue your juice fast through two whole days, fine. The longer you maintain your Juice Blitz, the more deep-cleansing your body can accomplish at a cellular level. But don't overdo it. Your body can't reverse the negative effects of years on a poor diet in a single week, or even a month. The Juice Blitz is intended to jump-start a process that it may take years to complete. It is not a way of life. You'll know how long you can maintain a juice fast because your body will tell you when it's over by making you overwhelmingly hungry!

As soon as you experience extreme pangs of hunger, break your fast. If, at any time while blitzing, you experience symptoms more serious than those listed under 'Trouble Shooting' (pages 215–16), consult your doctor or medical advisor. If you are contemplating a juice fast lasting longer than two or three days, it's a good idea to consult a health practitioner who is experienced in juice therapy before you begin.

The Plan

Before you start blitzing, do a little forward planning. You are going to need a fair quantity of fruits and vegetables, so make a list before you shop to ensure you remember everything. Where possible, always buy fruits and vegetables that have been grown organically, without the use of chemical fertilizers and pesticides. Often, organic produce doesn't look as good as the cheaper stuff that's displayed in the supermarket, but it is inherently better for you because none of its nutritional integrity has been compromised. People are waking up to the truth of this statement so rapidly that there is a shortage of organic produce across Europe and it might not be easy for you to locate a supplier, but it is quite definitely worth the effort.

Over the course of the weekend, your biggest enemy may well be boredom. Breaking from your usual dietary regime is never completely effortless and if you are bored you might well suffer hunger pangs and be tempted to start snacking. So find something to preoccupy your mind over the weekend. Read novels or watch videos; write letters or telephone friends you haven't seen for a while.

BLITZ ESSENTIALS:
THE EIGHT GREAT ELIMINATORS

Merry Belon

Melons go through the system faster than any other fruit and are therefore recommended by many juice experts to be drunk on their own. The key to the melon's efficacy is the exceptionally high water content of the flesh, while the nutrients are concentrated in the rind and skin, which can and should also be juiced. Some melons like honeydew and cantaloupes have waxy or netted skins which can be trimmed off with a decent vegetable peeler. Others, like watermelons, can be simply scrubbed, sliced to fit your juicer and put through the machine, seeds and all.

Melons in general and watermelons in particular are a perfect source of the fluids your body needs on a daily basis and a good source of B-complex vitamins, as well as being rich in vitamin C. There is an ever-growing profusion of melon varieties on the market, and it's fun to experiment with all of them. But melon juice can be a bit on the bland side. The addition of a handful of succulent summer berries will brighten it up considerably.

Berries are the one fruit that combines really well with melons and the array of flavours gives lots of scope for experimentation. In hot weather, a good tip is to freeze your berries before juicing them. Try Galia & Raspberry, Honeydew & Blackberry or the classic Watermelon & Strawberry:

*1 slice of watermelon, 3cm wide and cut into chunks to
fit your juicer*
*6 strawberries, washed and with their green stalks
removed*

Citrus Zinger

Whole citrus juice freshly-extracted using a centrifugal machine has a homogenized, creamy texture and tastes like sherbet. The pith of grapefruit is especially rich in bioflavonoids, which is hardly surprising since grapefruit juice tends to be the most bitter of the citrus family. Pink grapefruits are sweeter and juicier than plain yellow ones and you have to pay a premium price for them, but it's worth it. It's sometimes hard to get hold of good, juicy oranges but the Mandarin varieties, like tangerines, are a good substitute in the depths of winter.

The skin of citrus fruits is often waxed to preserve its shelf life and, therefore, should always be removed. Even a sliver of lemon peel put through your juicer can ruin the taste of your juice. Use lemons and limes sparingly, never adding more than half of either fruit to a glass of juice. The following recipe is a mélange of citrus spiked with ginger for an intriguing aftertaste. Feel free to vary it as you like:

1 orange
1 pink grapefruit
½ lemon or lime
1cm cube of ginger (optional)

Fab 5 Fruit Juice

You can vary the fruit content as you like and depending on what you are able to buy, you can substitute a clementine or satsuma for the tangerine, white grapes for red, and pineapple or mango for the peach. Apples and pears should be cut to fit your juicer and put through the machine, pips and all. Remove the stones from peaches and mangoes. Cut the fibrous skin from pineapples and slice them into long spears. This fruit mix is thick and frothy with a pleasant, balanced flavour that's especially good on a warm day when you might like to add some ice cubes to it and sip it slowly through a straw:

½ apple
½ pear
1 tangerine
A dozen red grapes
1 peach

Sweet Salvation

Sweet capsicums (peppers) produce a juice with amazing colour and fantastic flavour, but they also contain more vitamin C than oranges. Sadly, many peppers these days are grown for looks rather than flavour. Pick the ones with the deepest colour and wash them well before use. Freshly-made tomato juice bears little relation to the canned variety and reminds us of why these succulent, savoury fruit were once called love apples. Look for vine-ripened tomatoes, which have better flavour. This cocktail has a deep red-orange colour and can be a bit thick. Dilute it with the judicious addition of cucumber, which should be peeled before it is juiced unless it is organically grown.

1 *red or yellow pepper*
2 *ripe tomatoes (or 1 beef tomato)*
1–2 *carrots*
3*cm section of cucumber*

More Raw NRG

Like the plain Raw NRG cocktail in Recipes (p.305), More Raw is based on the crucial combination of carrot and apple, with green vegetable juices diluted by cucumber and celery. The juice extracted from green veggies is very powerful, both in its healthful properties and its taste. Spinach and watercress are invaluable for conditioning the entire digestive system thanks to the oxalic acid they contain, which helps to maintain the action of peristalsis. They are also amongst the best sources of vitamins C and E. Dandelion leaves are the first spring greens to sprout. They're an excellent source of calcium and potassium and the best known source of beta-carotene among the green vegetables. No wonder rabbits love them.

You will find the green juices a little strong at first, and will need to dilute them with cucumber and celery, but as you get used to the taste you can incorporate more leaves into your juices. When making this juice, put the ingredients through your juicer in this order and you'll end up with a greenish drink tinged with orange froth:

1 *small bunch of spinach or watercress (or dandelion)*
 leaves
1 *floret of broccoli*
3*cm section of cucumber*
2 *stalks of celery*
1 *apple*
3 *carrots*

Potassium Punch

This recipe is our tribute to N.W. Walker, the American raw food pioneer and proponent of natural healing who helped to develop the technique of juicing and was one of the first to write about the wonders of raw juice. A marvellous testament to the truth of the idea that you are what you eat, Dr Walker lived to the age of 106. An evangelist of detoxification, he would recommend to his patients that they drink his Raw Potassium Broth, although he would be the first to admit that most people don't find it as palatable as straight carrot juice or concoctions based on a carrot and apple mix.

In the words of the great man himself: 'The organic minerals and salts in this combination of raw potassium 'broth' embrace practically the entire range of those required by the body. Its effect in reducing excessive acidity in the stomach has been truly remarkable. There is probably no food more complete in every respect than this for the human organism.' So there you have it. We recommend that you drink at least a glass a day.

3 carrots
2 stalks celery
4–6 leaves of lettuce or winter greens
A handful of spinach or watercress (or dandelion) leaves
A few stalks of fresh coriander or parsley

Beet Treat

You have to be careful how you handle beetroot juice, which is most valuable for flushing the kidneys and enriching the blood, but can cause a dramatic cleansing action if taken in quantities of more than half a glass at a time. Cut the fibrous root off the bottom of your beets, but there's no need to peel them so long as they're thoroughly washed. You can include the leafy tops, too, if they are attached. The juice has a wonderful purple colour and an earthy, wholesome flavour. But don't over-do it. Take it from us that too much beet juice is liable to provoke a profoundly moving experience!

½ whole beetroot, including the leafy top if possible
2 carrots
1 apple
1 stalk of celery
3cm section of cucumber

Roots Soup

Root vegetables are the best source of thiamin, riboflavin, niacin and other water-soluble vitamins of the B complex and are abundant in trace elements. Their juices are thick, sweet and creamy and are complemented by the slightly aniseed flavour of fennel, which adds an intriguing dimension to this recipe. Fennel is a folk cure for heartburn in the Cajun country of Louisiana and a darned effective one at that. Dilute your root soup with cucumber juice, but if it's still too thick add a splash of spring water.

½ beetroot
1 medium-sized parsnip
1 sweet potato
½ bulb of fennel
5cm section of cucumber

Breathing & Brushing

The Juice Blitz will accelerate the detoxification of your body from within by flushing the bowels and kidneys, but these are only two of the routes by which toxins are expelled. Just as important are the lungs and the skin. While detoxing, it's important to pay special attention to both.

Breathing is the most fundamental process of life. It goes without saying that if you were deprived of oxygen, you'd expire within minutes, but no less crucial is the second half of the respiratory process: discarding carbon dioxide by breathing out. CO_2 is the poisonous by-product of oxidation and energy release in your cells which is carried back to the lungs in the blood and eliminated when you breathe out. At least that's how it *should* work but, since most of us use less than half of our breathing capacity, the system rarely functions as efficiently as it might. Learning to breathe properly is an elementary step towards reconditioning your body.

Most of us breathe with only the top half of our bodies, but proper breathing requires the use of the diaphragm, the muscle that separates the chest cavity from the abdomen. When you breathe correctly, the diaphragm contracts, allowing the lungs to expand and fill with air. During a single day, the average person will breathe in more than 11,000 litres of air. To make the best use of it all you must learn to breathe deeply, from the bottom up. You can ensure proper breathing and keep your lungs working well by taking a daily dose of aerobic exercise. In addition the following deep breathing exercise will be a great help:

1. Go outside into the fresh air, or open a window.
2. Stand with your feet slightly apart and your hands on your sides, touching your lower ribs just above the waist.
3. Inhale through your nose for the slow count of five and feel how your abdomen swells as you do so.
4. Continue to breathe in for another count of five, filling your lungs and expanding your rib cage.
5. Hold your breath for another count of five.

6. Exhale slowly through the mouth for the count of ten, noticing how your ribcage shrinks as you do so and pulling in with your abdominal muscles until you have expelled all the air.
7. Repeat this exercise four times.

Not only does breathing enable us to take in oxygen and expel CO_2, it also keeps the lymphatic system moving. These lymphatics are the body's sewage system: an elaborate network of microscopic channels that covers the whole body and is filled with a clear liquid called lymph. This is the medium by which nutrients are carried into the tissues of your body and metabolic waste is removed. There's more lymph in your body than blood and the lymphatic system is similar to the tiny capillaries of the pulmonary system, but with one vital difference. Whereas blood is pumped around your body by your heart, lymph has no pump and is only kept flowing by gravity and by muscular movement.

Get Moving

One of the best techniques for encouraging lymphatic drainage and spring-cleaning your body is known as skin brushing. It stimulates the movement of interstitial fluids and breaks down congestion in areas where the flow of lymph has become sluggish. Gentle yet powerful, it takes only five minutes in the morning or evening before your bath or shower and is both invigorating and pleasurable:

1. Use a natural-fibre brush with quite a long handle, or a loofah.
2. Begin at the tips of your shoulders and cover your whole body (except the head), working downwards, with long, smooth strokes over the shoulders, arms and trunk.
3. Starting at the feet, brush upwards over the legs and hips.

JUICE BLITZ: QUICK REFERENCE

The Night Before	Juice Blitz Day	Blitz Night & Morning After	The Rest of Your Life
For dinner, a glass of the More Raw NRG cocktail or Potassium Punch	Start with a melon or citrus juice and continue with fruit juices all day. Lunch: try a Beet Treat. Stick to vegetable juices (mixed with apple if desired) throughout the day.	Drink nothing but water after 8 o'clock. Start the next morning with fruit juice. Lunch: plenty of salad – your first meal after the Blitz should be 75 per cent raw foods.	The longer you maintain the Juice Blitz the more deep-cleansing your body will do. But don't overdo it. Break your fast as soon as you experience extreme pangs of hunger. The Juice Blitz is a jump-start for a process that may take years to complete. It is not a way of life but an invaluable tool.

TROUBLE SHOOTING

Most people experience no discomfort while blitzing their bodies with juice, but there are always exceptions. A small percentage of people, those whose systems are particularly toxic (and therefore most in need of detoxification) may experience one or more of the symptoms listed below. If this applies to you, don't let yourself be discouraged from continuing with the Juice Blitz for the full 36 hours. Remember that these complaints are not the signs of illness developing in your body, but of the toxins that cause illness leaving it. Recognize that they are temporary and will leave you feeling better than ever.

Bloating and/or Flatulence	This is quite common at the start of the Juice Blitz when you start consuming freshly-extracted fruit juices on an empty stomach. Its cleansing action will sluice the walls of your stomach and stir up accumulated food debris, causing wind. Look on it as the body girding itself for the work ahead.
Diarrhoea	What you may think of as diarrhoea probably isn't and certainly should not be anything to worry about. Raw juice will wash impacted faeces from your intestinal walls and expel it from the bowel in the form of loose, runny stools. This is highly beneficial and will leave you feeling lighter and renewed.

Headaches, Mood Swings, Irritability	These are all symptomatic of the chemical change in your body and are easily overcome if you understand them as a sign that the detoxification is starting to have its effect. Take a nap, go for a walk, or do the deep breathing exercise described above.
Tiredness and Boredom	The hard work of detoxifying your body requires a lot of energy, so it's quite natural to feel sleepy. Being bored is the result of inadequate preparation. Surely you can find something to amuse yourself with? Read, watch videos, play games. Just stay out of the pub.
Catarrh	Caught a cold? Actually, a copious discharge of mucus from your nasal passage rarely indicates a viral infection but is one of the classic ways in which the body eliminates stored toxins. So blow your snotty nose and be glad you're getting rid of them.
Perspiration	Your skin is the largest organ of elimination and the most direct route out of your body for a lot of toxins. Consequently, if you find that you perspire more heavily than usual while blitzing, particularly while you're asleep in bed, don't worry about it. If you are using the Juice Blitz to stop smoking, you are liable to lose quite a lot of fluid as your body takes the opportunity to expel the nicotine through the pores of the skin.

You need only go over your skin once for the brushing to be effective. Regular brushing will stimulate lymph-flow and unclog the pores of your skin. How firmly you press depends entirely on how well-toned your skin is. Go easy to begin with and become more vigorous as your skin gets fitter.

4
Body Building

Juice drinking works two kinds of magic on your body. The first is detoxification. Detox is central not only to healing illness but to protecting from degeneration as well as to regenerating and rejuvenating the body. That is why it forms the basis of every form of natural medicine in the world. The principle is simple: clean out the body and you raise vitality, strengthen its healing powers and set it free from the burden of chronic fatigue and heaviness that plagues the majority of men and women in industrialized countries these days. Once, detox itself was probably enough to heal and boost vitality. Now, as a result of widespread nutritional deficiencies, it is only half of what is called for. Now we need to look not only at how to *detox* the system but how to *rebuild* its metabolic pathways. We call this process body building.

Get a Life

As a result of the way we have depleted our foods of essential nutrients and distorted the vitamin and mineral balance in our bodies through chemical farming, heavy food processing, and long storage of our foods, most of us have nowhere near the optimal levels of vitamins, minerals and vital trace elements our bodies need to be superhealthy. Many nutrients – from vitamin B6 to the mineral zinc and the trace element silicon – must be present both in adequate amounts and in a good balance in order to stimulate the activity of enzymes on which every life process depends.

Your body cannot make its own minerals. It has to take them in, in a good balance, from the foods you eat. In addition to nitrogen, potassium and phosphorus, the body requires magnesium, manganese and calcium, selenium, zinc, copper, iodine, boron, molybdenum, vanadium and probably other elements as yet undiscovered.

Organic Magic

The organic matter in healthy soil is Nature's factory for biological activity. It is built up as a result of the breakdown of vegetable and animal matter by the soil's natural 'residents' – worms, bacteria and other useful microorganisms. The presence of these creatures in the right quantity and type gives rise to physical, chemical and biological properties that create fertility in our soils and make plants grown on them highly resistant to disease. When it comes to human health they do a lot more. The minerals and trace elements we need to trigger the metabolic processes *must* be in an organic form. That is, they need to be taken from living things like plant or animal foods. You cannot eat nails – inorganic iron – and expect to protect yourself from anaemia, or chew sand – inorganic silica – and be sure to get enough of the trace element to keep your nails and hair strong and help protect your bones from osteoporosis. It is the organic matter in soils that enables plants grown on them to transform inorganic iron and silica into the organic form which is taken up by the vegetables and fruits, grains and legumes grown on them. Organic methods of farming help protect against significant distortions in mineral balances – that is from an increase in one or more mineral elements which can alter the availability of others and undermine health. No such protection is available when foods are chemically grown.

Making Do

The deficiencies we are developing through eating chemically grown and processed foods have brought metabolic distortions in their wake – such as degenerative diseases, early ageing, and emotional disturbances like depression and anxiety. These kinds of deficiencies cannot easily be corrected. Popping the latest multi-mineral tablet from your corner pharmacy or healthfood store won't do it. Daily juicing will.

Nutrients in foods exist in complex synergy and affect each other. They interact and work together in your body. The balance of bio-available minerals and trace elements needed in the body for peak well-being is infinitely more complex than vitamin fanatics would have us believe. This is where raw juices really come into their own. To restore biochemical balance once it has been disturbed, you need a continual supply of the vitamins and minerals as well as other health-enhancing substances that are found in fresh vegetables and fruits and in green plants such as seaweeds, spirulina, chlorella, barley grass or alfalfa.

Perfect Synergy

Recent research has focused on seeking out and identifying specific nutrients and compounds – called phytochemicals – that are present within common foods and that appear to act naturally to prevent cancer and other diseases. Thanks to the particular balance of amino acids, enzymes, polysaccharides and other compounds they contain, such foods as garlic, liquorice, and green compounds like green barley, spirulina, chlorella and many other fresh foods have the ability to turn on the human immune system. Some contain *isoflavones* and *protease inhibitors* (see p.222) which are capable of breaking down layers surrounding foreign proteins, including tumours. Others are rich in *phyto-sterols* (see below), useful in protecting both men and women from reproductive damage by herbicides and pesticides (which act as oestrogen-mimics or *xenoestrogens* to lower sperm count in men and encourage PMS, osteoporosis, endometriosis and fibroids in women).

Blinkered Nutrition

One of the problems with most of the information that is handed out through the media and books on nutrition is that it is highly fragmented. You hear talk about a specific vitamin or mineral and how we should take more of it, about cholesterol or protein or fibre. We seem to have become obsessed in recent years with breaking everything down and looking at the effects of specific ingredients on our bodies. We have forgotten how to see the wood for the trees. It is not just the ingredient – a particular vitamin or mineral or compound – in a vegetable that can do us good. It is the synergy of nature, in which the whole is far greater than the sum of its parts.

Protective Compounds

In fresh fruits and vegetables, phyto-chemicals come in a total package. Here are some of the most important of the specific ingredients so far identified:

saponins: these have anti-oxidant properties and as such help prevent changes to the cells' DNA (our genetic coding) associated with premature ageing and the development of cancer. Research shows that cancer of the colon is much lower in populations where there is a high dietary intake of saponins.

phyto-sterols: these plant hormones include such chemicals as *stigmasterol* and *ergosterol* which are little absorbed in the digestive system. They pass on to

221

the colon where they help prevent damage from the cancer-producing breakdown products from cholesterol. Some phyto-sterols are also weak oestrogenic compounds capable of binding with oestrogen receptor sites in both male and female bodies, protecting against reproductive problems that develop as a result of exposure to xenoestrogens. Many phyto-sterols also help protect against premature ageing of the skin and skin cancer as well as prostate troubles, PMS and menopausal miseries.

phenolic acids: these anti-oxidants help prevent damage to cellular DNA associated with premature ageing and the development of degenerative diseases.

protease inhibitors: these compounds help protect against the damaging effects of toxins in the body and against radiation and free radical damage. In laboratory studies protease inhibitors have been shown to inhibit cancers of the mouth, pancreas, lung, colon and digestive tract. Unfortunately protease inhibitors – which exist in good quantities in many common wholesome foods including potatoes, eggs, and grains – are greatly destroyed by cooking. In many raw vegetables, however, they are in rich supply.

omega-3 fatty acids: these are essential fatty acids which, when unadulterated by heating or processing and taken fresh, have been shown to protect against cancer and heart disease. They also play important roles in the manufacture of hormones in the body and are found in good quantities in flaxseeds or linseeds, in sprouted seeds and grains which you can use for juicing, and in some of the special green foods such as spirulina.

isoflavones: these are plant hormones which carry strong anti-cancer properties, particularly in relation to cancers of the reproductive system such as prostate cancer, cervical cancer, ovarian cancer, endometrial cancer and breast cancer. The molecular structure of isoflavonoids is very close to that of the oestrogens, but they are only one hundred-thousandth as potent as the body's oestrogens and oestrogens given in the form of drugs. Eating foods or making juices of foods rich in the isoflavones can help protect both men and women from xenoestrogens in the environment. Japanese researchers have shown that the weak oestrogenic effect of isoflavones can relieve – often even completely eliminate – the negative symptoms associated with PMS and menopause.

Plant compounds play an important, if not yet fully understood, part in restoring the kind of biochemical balance that the body's metabolic processes need to function smoothly. You need only examine a couple of common vegetables to see just how powerful the protective, restoring plant compounds they contain can be.

Caring Carrot

Carrots are unbelievably rich in anti-oxidant and cancer-preventive compounds. The most well known of these is beta-carotene. This naturally occurring anti-oxidant has become famous in recent years as a safe-to-take precursor to vitamin A – something that your body can turn into vitamin A as needed. But beta-carotene is only the most well-researched of the carotenoids. Scientists are now discovering many others which appear to have equal if not greater health-supporting abilities. A high consumption of foods containing carotenoids has been shown to lower the incidence of lung, pancreas and prostate cancer. Even cancer among cigarette smokers is lower among people with carotinoid-rich diets. So much is this true that smokers on carotinoid-poor diets are four times more likely to get cancer than those who consume the carotinoids in even one carrot a day. Think how much more you get when you drink a full glass of fresh carrot juice each day. Carotinoids are by no means the only goodies in carrot juice, nor are carrots the only place that you will find good quantities of them. Spirulina – which is a wonderful green additive to juices – is ultra-rich in carotinoids, as are winter marrow, yams and other green vegetables.

Carrots also contain other fabulous health-boosting friends such as MOP – a little compound with an amazing ability to help repair DNA. Damage to DNA is the central cause of degeneration and premature ageing in the body. Prevent it and you can prevent early ageing. That is where MOP comes in. MOP actually tucks itself in between the base pairs of DNA molecules and repairs damage that has occurred. Scientists experimenting with MOP have found that they can take damaged white blood cells from people, add MOP to them and then put the white blood cells back into the body in perfect shape. Parsnips are also rich in MOP and mix well with carrot juice.

Green Glory

There are an amazing thirty-three cancer-preventive compounds in fresh broccoli. These include beta-carotene and indole-3-carbinol which have the ability to counteract many of the chemicals which pollute our environment – such as the *nitrosamines* which are known to cause cancer. (Nitrosamines are formed when nitrites are used to preserve and colour meat.) Indole-3-carbinol not only prevents cancer but also helps prevent other degenerative diseases as well as premature ageing. A cup full of broccoli or one of the other dark greens in a glass of carrot and apple juice once a day delivers 165 per cent of the recommended daily allowance for vitamin C, 40 per cent for vitamin A and 20 per cent for calcium.

Natural Healing

Most people have never heard of the indoles or saponins or any of the other fresh food compounds that can encourage radiant health – although volumes have been written about their virtues in scientific literature. Even more esoteric is the knowledge about how juices made from fresh raw foods enhance health not from a *chemical* point of view but rather from an *energetic* one. World experts in natural healing have made remarkable use of raw foods and their juices to help the body eliminate cancer from its system, cure migraine, rejuvenate, and improve athletic performance.

Back to Basics

Human evolution is a slow process. For hundreds of generations our ancestors lived on wild foods gathered and eaten raw. Our genes appear to be specially adapted to dealing with raw foods. The famous Swiss physician Max Bircher-Benner and the German Max Gerson used living foods not only to support the human organism's healing but also to heighten vitality as well as to regenerate and rejuvenate the body as a whole. By incorporating a good percentage of live foods – fresh vegetables, raw seeds and nuts, fresh sprouted grains and seeds and especially fresh vegetable juices – in your diet you can help rebalance hormones, stabilize moods, clear and rejuvenate skin, shed excess fat stores and transform your emotional and spiritual outlook on life.

More than fifty years ago the distinguished Viennese doctor Hans Eppinger discovered that a high-raw way of eating leads to increased cellular respiration. It does this in a number of ways, creating a kind of positive feedback loop which leads to heightened cell metabolism. It eliminates accumulated wastes and toxins from cells and tissues. It supplies the level of nutrients essential for optimal cell function. And, perhaps most important of all, it heightens the micro-electrical tensions associated with cell vitality so that even cells in a particularly sluggish and neglected system are revitalized. They become better able to burn calories in the presence of oxygen and to produce energy efficiently both for overall vitality and for carrying out the housekeeping on which the health of your body depends.

Micro-Electrics

Capillaries are minute blood vessels which form a vast network of microcirculation throughout your body. It is their responsibility to deliver oxygen-rich blood for it to be used by the cells. So important are these fine vessels that nature has supplied you with incredible lengths of them. If you were to attach all the capillaries in your body end to end they would measure some 60,000 miles in length – more than twice around the world. The condition of your body as a whole depends to a great extent on the state of your capillaries. As the arbitrators of cell nutrition, respiration and elimination, capillaries carry nutrients and oxygen around your body. Each of them has tiny 'pores' which allow plasma (but not red blood cells) to seep through and pass into the body fluid. This is how nutrients are delivered and wastes eliminated from tissues. Without good microcirculation, metabolism cannot take place efficiently. That is why the capillaries play a vital part in the successful elimination of excess fat deposits with all their stored toxins.

Unfortunately, over the years the capillaries of people living on the average western diet (with its excessive fats, proteins and refined and processed food) become twisted, distended and highly porous. When this happens, proteins seep through and deposit themselves between the tissues and the capillary walls, where they interfere with proper oxygen exchange and impede nutrient delivery and waste elimination. This can gradually starve cells, tissues and organs of all they need to function properly and can also lower cellular metabolic activity. In this deprived condition the entire organism (i.e. your body) is predisposed to degenerative illness and to rapid ageing. A Juice High lifestyle, drinking three or four glasses of freshly made juice, at least two of which are primarily vegetable juices, helps restore normal microcirculation. This in turn heightens metabolism, keeping your weight down and maintaining a high level of energy.

Dynamic Tensions

The interchange of chemicals and energy between the microcirculation and the cells takes place through two thin membranes and a fine interstitial space. And it happens only because the cells and capillaries have what is known as 'selective capacity'. This means they are able to absorb the substances they need and to reject what is harmful or unnecessary for metabolic processes. This selective capacity is the result of antagonistic chemical and micro-electrical tensions in the cells and tissues of all living systems. When you suffer from a chronic degenerative condition or when metabolism is lowered these micro-electrical tensions are drastically reduced. The stronger the tensions – the more intense these antagonisms – the healthier and more vital your body will be and the more efficiently it will be able to burn off stored fat and eliminate toxicity. The chronic fatigue and lowered metabolism which typically occur in women as they grow older – particularly if they have been on and off low-calorie slimming regimes over the years – is accompanied by a decrease in chemical and micro-electrical tensions and a loss of selective capacity. Cell reproduction slows down, capillary walls are weakened and there is a gradual build-up in the interstitial spaces of a sticky 'marsh' derived from excess waste products. This marsh, or tissue sludge, impedes biochemical processes including the production and balancing of hormones and tends to lower metabolism even further, impairing the efficient elimination of wastes by the lymph system.

The lymph nodes, which are located in the groin and under the arm and the neck, filter the lymphatic fluid to remove impurities and dead cells; they are also a place where antibodies, which fight infection or toxins, are made. After purification at the nodes, the fluid is returned to the blood. However, when the lymph system becomes clogged or does not eliminate properly the body can become seriously burdened with toxicity.

Excess toxicity is the common factor in the development of degenerative diseases such as arthritis, cancer, heart disease and diabetes as well as early ageing, the development of persistent cellulite in women's bodies and the tendency to store and to maintain a high level of fat deposits in both men and women.

Increase Selective Capacity

Eppinger and another German scientist, Karl Eimer, showed why drinking live juices and eating lots of fresh raw vegetables can change all this. They steadily *increase* selective capacity by heightening electrical potentials between tissue cells and capillary blood. This improves the ability of your capillaries to regulate the transport of nutrients. It also helps detoxify the system, removing any sticky marsh of waste products that may be present. A way of eating that is high in living foods and their juices, where say 50 per cent of what you eat is taken raw, together with regular exercise, breaks through that vicious circle of fatigue replacing it with a well-functioning metabolism which makes detoxification and the rebuilding of the body's metabolism a steady, straightforward occurrence.

Drink lots of raw juices and choose the rest of your foods from wholesome natural products such as grains and pulses, sea plants, fresh vegetables, fresh locally-grown fruits, and tofu, and you will notice a dramatic improvement in how you look and feel and function within the first couple of weeks. But it will be several weeks before the burden of toxicity which you have been carrying has fully cleared, and it will probably be a few months before even deeper benefits begin to show themselves. By then any pre-existing subclinical vitamin or mineral deficiencies should clear up completely. So be patient. Your body has a quite magnificent ability to heal itself and to excel at being superhealthy, but this doesn't happen overnight.

5
High Life

The Juice Blitz is a first-rate, quick-fix detox regime that gives you an intimation of the Juice High lifestyle. Once you've experienced its clear-headed benefits, you'll want to take it further. The next step, as we've just seen, is *body building*, using raw juices to replenish lost vitamins, mineral and trace elements, and to help prevent degenerative diseases as well as energize, regenerate and rejuvenate your body. The High Life Diet will give you all the support you need to carry on the good work.

High Life is an exciting, delicious food style for the future which satisfies the senses and fuels the body so that it functions at peak efficiency on an on-going basis. Its high raw food content and its dependence on wholesome *real* food – instead of the ersatz packaged stuff that these days masquerades as food – provides the kind of high quality nutrition you require to feel fully alive. On page 243 we give you a High Life Ten-Day Programme which can be followed as a short-term, quick-fix regime to enhance your overall health. More significantly, the diet can be used as the blueprint for a permanent change in the way you eat to build and sustain optimum well-being.

The Big Idea

There is nothing complicated about High Life – just a few simple principles that determine what to eat and when to eat it. Breakfast is raw juice with green supplements and as much whole fruit as you want. Try to make lunch the main meal of the day. It begins with a green drink and is built around a terrific Trio Salad (see p. 315) composed of one root vegetable, one fruit vegetable, and one leafy vegetable. What else? A good source of protein such as tofu, eggs, steamed or grilled fish or chicken – preferably cooked without the skin – and organic meat.

Dinner should be light. Perhaps a glass of raw juice followed by a bowl of home-made vegetable soup spiked with sea vegetables for extra minerals and flavour, or a crunchy salad with some wholegrain bread.

It may not be practicable for you to take a long break in the middle of the day, but whenever possible make lunch your largest meal. This is when you most need energy for the day.

If you get into the habit of eating light in the evening, you'll find that you will sleep far better at night. Soon, you will probably find that you are sleeping a lot less, too. When your body is detoxified and functioning efficiently, you will sleep more soundly. Because the sleep you get on the High Life diet is more restful, you need less of it.

Cut out Coffee

We love coffee, adore the stuff. The kind of coffee we particularly like is real strong, dark and potent espresso of the kind that gives you a better buzz than amphetamine sulphate. The comparison with an illegal drug is apposite, since trimethyl xanthine – caffeine – is also habit-forming and its overuse can lead to headaches, insomnia, nervousness, and anxiety. Like speed, coffee gives you a quick lift and the illusion of energy, only to let you crash a few hours later in need of another caffeine injection to keep going. Consequently, while we still drink coffee occasionally, we're careful not to let it become a daily habit.

Have you ever had to work late, perhaps revising for an exam, and kept yourself going with endless cups of coffee? If so, you'll be familiar with that wired mental state in which your thoughts are racing, but you just can't seem to get them into any sort of comprehensible order. Caffeine stimulates your nervous system and makes you feel alert, but tests have demonstrated that in reality the drug causes confusion and nervousness. Rather than help you concentrate, too much coffee has the effect of disconnecting you from your instincts and, in extreme cases, can provoke a psychotic reaction. In fact, if you need a clear head and the stamina to keep studying for hours on end, the best thing to keep you going is a glass of raw juice.

Some people use coffee as a laxative, but while it's certainly effective at moving the bowels, caffeine has a strongly adverse effect on the digestive system as a whole. Tea is not much better for you. Even if you've always been a committed tea drinker, after a couple of weeks of living the Juice High life you'll find you don't miss it. Then, you will appreciate an occasional cup of Rosie Lee or powerful shot of espresso as one of life's simple pleasures rather than a matter of addiction.

Table Manners

Eating and drinking are usually seen as correlated activities. We tend to do both at meal times, simultaneously, sluicing chewed food down our oesophagus with abandon while raising the next forkful to our lips. Too often we eat on the run, cramming food into our mouths and washing it down with great gulps of drink. We know that eating like this isn't very dignified and probably isn't too good for the digestion, but we do it anyway. Then, when we get indigestion, we complain that there must have been something wrong with the food rather than the way we consumed it.

To live the High Life, however, you are going to have to do something about sloppy table manners. The High

Life Diet requires you to become more discriminating about what you eat, and you must also be more fastidious about the way you eat it. While we occasionally enjoy a glass of wine or two over dinner, drinking a lot at meal times is not a good idea – for two reasons. First, drinking tends to make you chew your food less thoroughly than you should. Second, fluids dilute the saliva in your mouth and the gastric juices in your stomach, rendering them ineffective at breaking down the improperly chewed food.

Accompany your meals with a glass of spring water if you wish, but just the one. Sip it slowly between mouthfuls, to clear your palate. Take the time to chew your food thoroughly before swallowing it. Don't talk with your mouth full and don't leap up from the table as soon as you're finished, but take a calm minute to let your food settle.

Just Juice

You'll notice how a glass of raw juice tends to fill you up, as if it were a meal in itself. In fact, considering the nutritional value of raw juice, it *is* a meal in itself and should be consumed on its own. Raw juice is easy to digest, but it still has to pass through your stomach to be assimilated in your intestines and anything eaten at the same time will only slow its passage. If taken on an empty stomach, raw juice will take no more than 20 minutes to pass through your stomach. Therefore, make it a rule not to eat or drink anything for at least that length of time after downing a glass of raw juice.

The living enzymes in raw juice assist the digestion process and the neutralizing effect of raw juice upon the internal environment of your body will provide the ideal conditions for food to be properly digested. Consequently, raw juice makes the ideal aperitif, or first course of a meal. At dinner parties, your guests will be delighted and amazed by being offered a glass of freshly-extracted raw juice in place of the soup. Just remember (and tell your friends!) to sip your juice slowly, mixing it with the saliva in your mouth, and try to wait half an hour before moving on to the main course.

With fruit juices, the half hour rule is slightly different, but even more important. Fruit juices pass through your stomach really quickly, in 10 or 15 minutes, so long as there is no food in the way. If the exit to your intestines is blocked by half-digested food, the fruit juice will be trapped in your stomach where it will start to ferment, causing bloating and flatulence. For this reason, fresh fruit and fruit juices should only be consumed on an empty stomach. In order to allow your body to complete its work of elimination before you start to burden your system once more with food, resolve to consume nothing but freshly-extracted fruit juices right up until midday.

One Green Glass

Fruit juices are fabulous, naturally, and we have yet to meet someone who wasn't beguiled by their first taste of Carrot & Apple. These are the easiest juices to accept, but they are far from being the most beneficial. In Chapter Seven, we explain more about the amazing and as yet unexplained but awesomely powerful health-promoting factors in the juices of green, leafy vegetables. To really live the High Life, you must incorporate more green vegetables into your diet. That's not a radical statement; everybody is saying it, from Government agencies to your mum.

To derive the maximum benefit from your juicer, therefore, you must make full use of the pungent and powerfully-flavoured dark green juices extracted from such vegetables as spinach, broccoli and cabbage. These all contain an abundance of micro-nutrients, enzymes and trace elements that are easily denatured by heat and totally destroyed by cooking. By juicing them, we are able to extract most of the essential goodness of raw vegetables and supply our bodies with unadulterated, natural green nutrition.

The snag is that these green juices tend to be something of an acquired taste. They are too strong to be drunk straight and must be diluted with blander and more watery salad vegetables, like cucumber and celery. Cucumbers are rich in minerals, but are mostly water; the juice is a strong diuretic and the best skin toner we know of. Unfortunately, the bright green specimens you see in the supermarket have often been sprayed with pesticides and waxed to preserve their appeal. Unless you're sure your cuke is organic, peel it. Celery has a mildly salty flavour and is also good for the complexion. It's often a bit muddy at the root, so wash each stalk thoroughly before you put it through the juicer.

Make it a rule that you will drink at least one glass of green juice each day. That doesn't mean you have to stick exclusively to green ingredients, just make sure that they form a good percentage of what you juice. Use a base of carrot and apple, as we do in the Raw NRG mix (see p. 305) and gradually include more and more green, as in the More Raw NRG cocktail (see p. 209). Generally speaking, the darker green the colour of your juice, the more good it's going to do you.

Less is More

Busy people tend to skip meals. They get caught up in their work, rushing to meet deadlines, and neglect to eat. This is by no means a bad thing, since being slightly hungry tends to make us more alert and creative. In fact it would be fine if, once their work was done, these busy people took their time to prepare and consume a properly-balanced meal like the ones we suggest in the Recipe section (see pages 315–22). But busy people don't tend to do that. They're too busy. So they live on convenience food.

People who want to lose weight in a hurry also tend to skip meals. They think that by doing without lunch they can forgo a few calories and maybe shed a few ounces. It might work, too, except that too often they find themselves craving confectionery in the middle of the afternoon, or being irresistibly drawn to the soft drinks machine in the corner of the office. There's nothing wrong with skipping meals, so long as you don't try to compensate for the meal you missed by eating (or drinking) junk later on.

Not only is there nothing wrong with skipping meals, it can be positively good for you. Increasingly, scientific evidence suggests that longevity can be significantly increased by a diet that contains a high level of essential nutrients, but about a third fewer calories than are conventionally thought necessary to maintain 'normal' body weight. A glass of raw juice is the ultimate dietary supplement and the perfect replacement for a bulky meal because it is nutrient-dense, but calorie-lean. Have a glass of raw juice instead of lunch and you will probably have plenty of energy to last you through until teatime. If you miss lunch and come home starving, don't dive into the biscuit barrel or raid the fridge for something to snack on before dinner. Make yourself a glass of raw juice instead.

Where's the Fibre?

Nutritionally, raw juice is excellent, but it is deficient in one department. Of all the insoluble fibre contained within the fruits and vegetables you juice, none of it goes into the glass. It's precisely because all the fibre has been extracted that raw juice is so effective in delivering essential nutrients to the body, but mankind cannot live by juice alone. Plenty of fibre in your diet is a prerequisite for good health and proper elimination, because it provides the muscles in your digestive tract with something solid to work with and acts as a peristaltic broom, collecting faecal matter in your colon and propelling it to the bowels. Fibre, as they say, keeps you regular.

The best source of fibre is raw fruits and vegetables, whole grains and pulses, of which you'll find plenty in the High Life Diet. Raw juice does contain *some* soluble dietary fibre, but all the insoluble cellulose fibre ends up with the pulp. We're frequently asked what to do with the pulp left over from juicing and there are various ways in which it can be used.

Pulp Facts

Many of the books on juicing don't tell you what to do with the pulp. The pulp is important. The average person on a Western diet gets only 10–25 grammes of fibre a day, whereas our ancestors were used to 35–60 grammes a day, so the more fibre you can use from your juicing the better.

There are all sorts of things you can do with vegetable and fruit pulps, but there is one principle you have to know. Either use the pulp right away in whatever dish you want to make – salad, sorbet, meat loaf, sauce, or a poultice (more about this in a minute) – or freeze it. It is easy to freeze fruit and vegetable pulps in plastic bags which you can then use at your leisure.

Cheap Beauty

There are all sorts of wonderful external poultices you can make from vegetable and fruit pulps. The pulps of kiwi fruit, pineapple, papaya and mango are wonderful for refining skin – in fact they are the natural source of the AHA fruit acids that you pay a fortune for in expensive skin creams. Simply apply the pulp to your skin, leave it on for ten minutes and rinse off. Because these tropical fruits contain proteolytic enzymes they will quite literally digest the dead skin cells on the surface of your skin, leaving it smoother, fresher, and regenerated.

The pulp from potatoes and cucumber are very useful as eye compresses. Simply place between two pieces of cheesecloth or cotton and lay over your closed eyelids while you rest for ten or fifteen minutes. This takes away bags from under the eyes, and minimises black circles.

Pumpkin, cucumber, carrot and marrow pulps are great for calming skin inflammations, whether they be eczema rash or sunburn. They are very cooling to the body and can be useful when you have a mild fever. Place in a compress in between two pieces of cotton on the forehead or just over the liver.

Pulps make great additions to salads too. You can also use pulp to stuff courgettes, tomatoes, marrows, even twice-baked potatoes. (Bake a potato, take out the inner part of the potato, mix with vegetable pulp, season with salt, pepper, and a little olive oil. Put back in the oven, sprinkled with some chopped spring onions, and rebake for fifteen minutes.) Pulp also goes well in pasta salads. And you can make wonderful soups by juicing vegetables, then mixing some of the juice back into the pulp and eating it immediately.

Delicious Sweets

You can use the pulp of fruits to bake beautiful sweet breads and rolls or to make carrot cake. Fruit pulps, fresh or frozen, such as apricot, pear, apple and peach, are great things to add to porridge, muesli or cereals along with a dash of cinnamon, nutmeg or cardamom. They bring a natural sweetness to the cereal without your ever having to add honey or sugar. You can also mix fruit pulps with yoghurt, cottage cheese or tofu, adding a little unsulphured blackstrap molasses or maple syrup to make delicious shakes. Finally, you can use fruit pulps warmed up a little to make delicious toppings for toast, pancakes or muffins. You can even mix them in with minced lamb or beef, pork or chicken, to make delicious high-fibre patties. Any pulp left over that you don't have a use for makes fabulous compost. You don't even have to wait for it to rot down; just spread it around your garden.

Here are a few of our favourite pulp recipes but do develop your own. You would be surprised how much you can get out of pulp.

Coleslaw

2 cups cabbage pulp
2 cups carrot pulp
1 cup apple pulp
1 tbsp cider vinegar
3 tbsp olive oil
2 tbsp chopped parsley
A handful of chopped spring onions

Mix all the pulps together, stir in the vinegar and olive oil and garnish with the parsley and spring onion.

Pasta Salad

1 bag wholegrain pasta of your choice
3 tbsp carrot pulp
3 tbsp celery pulp
3 tbsp tomato pulp
3 tbsp cauliflower pulp
salt and pepper to taste
1 tsp oregano
2 squeezed cloves garlic
4 tbsp olive oil

Cook the pasta and chill. Add the rest of the ingredients, mix and serve.

Yummy Carrot Cake

1 cup cold-pressed sesame oil or olive oil
3 cups carrot pulp
1 cup apple pulp
1 cup honey
½ cup blackstrap molasses
1 tsp pure vanilla extract
3 eggs
3 cups wholegrain flour
1½ tsp baking soda
2 tsp nutmeg
1 cup raisins

Mix the pulps and oil together, add the honey, molasses, vanilla and eggs and mix together well. Sift together the dry ingredients and add to the mixture, stir until blended. Add the raisins, pour into an oiled baking pan and bake for one hour at 180°C (350°F) Gas 4.

Blueberry Muffins

3 cups carrot pulp
1½ cups pineapple pulp
1 cup honey
3 eggs
1 cup cold-pressed sesame oil or extra-virgin olive oil
1 tbsp vanilla
3 cups wholegrain flour
1 tbsp baking soda
1 tsp nutmeg
1½ cups fresh or frozen whole blueberries

Mix the carrot and the pineapple pulp together, add the honey, eggs, oil and vanilla and mix. Sift together the dry ingredients and add to the mixture. Add the blueberries and stir in gently. Pour into muffin papers or greased muffin tins. Bake for 45 minutes at 180°C (350°F) Gas 4.

Pulp Sorbet

Collect about three cups of pulp from any sweet fruit – peaches, apples, cherries, pears, apricots, pine-apple, raspberries, strawberries. Freeze in an ice-cube tray and when frozen put into a food processor with 4 ripe bananas and blend to the consistency of sorbet. Serve immediately.

Fruit Sauce

Take 1 cup of pulp from any sweet fruit, blend together with 2 tbsp honey or organic maple syrup and serve on toast or pancakes or over ice cream.

Total Juicing

Conventional juicers, whether they be centrifugal juicers or extruding juicers, all separate the juice from the pulp. You then have the option of using the pulp (which is what we strongly recommend since it is full of vitamins and minerals) or throwing it away. However, there is a whole new approach to juicing which is worth getting into. It is called molecular juicing, or *total juicing*, and it requires a totally different piece of equipment from the machine you use for ordinary juice making.

Total juicing is a way of juicing the entire vegetable or fruit, from which you discard nothing. It actually pulverizes the fruit or vegetable to such a fine degree that you are able to absorb the nutrients almost immediately. This form of juicing is wonderful for anyone who has a digestive problem, for babies, for anyone who wants to get large quantities of fibre – for example, someone who is slimming – and for anyone whose digestion is less than perfect.

For total juicing you need a very strong machine. Conventional blenders are not capable of molecular or total juicing. They will give you a mush that is highly unpleasant. You need to remember that total juicing takes a lot more skill in what you mix with what, as if you mix combinations of fruits and vegetables together indiscriminately you can end up with a mess that tastes disgusting.

Total juicing is also a wonderful way of increasing the fibre in your diet. Many important ingredients in a fruit or vegetable are actually left in the fibre (and that's another reason why we urge you strongly not to discard the pulp). For instance, when you extract the juice from an orange you get approximately 30IU of beta-carotene, but 30 more are discarded in the pulp. With a carrot, you get 14,000IU of carotene in the juice but another 9800IU remain in the fibre. With total juicing you get them all.

The juice you produce by placing your fruits or vegetables cut into convenient sized pieces into a molecular or total juicer is not as sweet as that which is extracted from one of the more conventional juicers. Hence total juicers can be a good thing for people with blood sugar problems, since occasionally they may find that the sweetness of carrot and apple, for instance, is such that it stimulates the pancreas to produce too much insulin.

Total juices have a thicker, smoother texture, a totally different feeling in the mouth to the juices which come out of ordinary juice extractors. Occasionally you might find you want to add a little sweetening to total juices and this is best done in the form of maple syrup or natural unheated honey. You will probably also need to add a little water or some ice cubes in order to give a bit more liquid for the pulverizing process to take place properly.

Soups & Sprouts

If you have a blender capable of total juicing, first make your vegetable or fruit juice in the ordinary way and then use it as an additive in your total juicing. So, if you have made some carrot juice, use it as a base for making beautiful vegetable soups (see Recipes, pages 320–22). Similarly you can use fruit juices as a base for making fruit frappés by mixing together whole fruits – peaches, apricots, berries – in the blender with the juice that you have made from your conventional juicer.

Total juicing is a great way of using sprouted alfalfa and mung beans. You simply take any vegetable or fruit juice, pour it into your total juicer and add a handful of your sprouts. Blend and drink immediately. The fibre in sprouted seeds is wonderful and it's a great way of getting the very best of both ways of juicing.

A total juicer is thus an ideal way of making green drinks. After preparing a vegetable or fruit juice in an ordinary juicer, pour into the blender and add green supplements such as fresh green beetroot leaves, kale, spinach or dandelion. You can also use the same method to add powdered wheat or barley grass to fresh juices. We always try to use organic fruits and vegetables for juicing just to be sure that we are protected from any intake of pesticides or herbicides.

HIGH LIFE TEN-DAY PROGRAMME

Now let's see what High Life looks like. Here are the basic guidelines for ten days to reorientate your eating habits permanently.

- Have juice for breakfast plus a green supplement either on its own or together with some fruit.

- Remember to *chew your juices and drink your food*. In other words, sip your juices slowly so they have a chance to mix with the saliva in the mouth to get the full benefit of everything that is in them, and chew your foods, until they turn into liquids.

- Avoid eating between meals since this slows down the

A DAY ON THE HIGH LIFE DIET

Begin the day with a cup of hot or cold spring water with the juice of half a lemon and a little honey or organic maple syrup if desired.

Throughout the day drink as much spring water as you like. If you are hungry between meals have another glass of juice, preferably green.

Breakfast

Large glass fresh raw fruit juice – apple, orange, grape, grapefruit etc, or a recipe of your choice. To this add either some green leaves such as dandelion, beetroot, spinach, the juice from one of the cereal grasses, or a teaspoon to a tablespoon of one of the cereal grass supplements such as green barley, stirred into your glass of juice. You can drink more than one juice (with or without the extra green) and you can also have a piece of fruit or a bunch of grapes and as much herb tea as you like, sweetened with a little honey or maple syrup.

Main Meal

If at all possible make this meal at lunchtime since you will digest your food better and sleep better if you eat light in the evening.

Large glass of fresh, raw vegetable juice, choose any mixture you like – carrot, raw beetroot, celery, cucumber, cabbage, tomato, spinach etc – or one of the recipes on pages 289–314.

A big salad – ideally one of the Trio Salads (see Recipes) together with some grilled fish, lamb's liver, free-range chicken, game, a tofu dish or an omelette.

Steamed or wok-fried vegetables.

Herb tea or coffee substitute.

Light Meal

Glass of fresh vegetable or fruit juice.

A salad or light soup.

Several slices of wholegrain bread or a bowl of live muesli.

Herb tea or coffee substitute.

stomach's emptying and encourages food that is still in the stomach to ferment, as well as creating false appetite. If you are hungry have a glass of fresh juice or lots of spring water between meals.

- Try to leave four to five hours between meals. This is the time your body needs in order to efficiently and completely digest its previous meal.

- Make meal times a pleasure.

- Drink as much water as you like, virtually the more the better. But don't drink water with meals – give yourself twenty minutes water-free before a meal and half an hour afterwards.

- Try to take your main meal at lunch and the light meal in the evening. This is an ideal way to live since you sleep much deeper and better if you don't eat heavily at night. However, you must suit your eating to your lifestyle and when you have to have a main meal at night, enjoy it.

6

Quick Fix

Because raw juice is the richest available source of vitamins, minerals and enzymes it is the best possible tonic for promoting all-round health and general well-being. Most people who embrace the Juice High lifestyle find that the minor complaints that used to irritate them fade away as the body rebalances itself and they become accustomed to feeling perfectly fine, all of the time. The key to building and sustaining an indomitable physiology, one which is strong, focused and invulnerable to illness, is the consumption of the broadest possible range of juices. However, each juice has specific therapeutic properties and this chapter shows how you can use raw juice to treat a range of common complaints.

Modern medical science tends to have a nuts and bolts approach in prescribing drugs to treat the symptoms of illness, frequently without paying attention to the underlying causes of the condition. Natural health practitioners try to take a holistic view, seeing the body as a complete organism with many parts, all of which must operate synergistically for the whole being to be healthy. Illness is the result of disharmony, or a chemical imbalance in the body caused by nutritional deficiency.

Here are our suggestions as to which foods you should eat (and which ones you should avoid) in order to alleviate the misery of a number of all-too-common complaints. Our suggestions are followed, in each case, by a list of appropriate juice recipes that you'll find in the Recipe Section which begins on page 289. Most of the conditions described below will respond rapidly when you drink the recommended juices, but do remember that these are only recommendations, not prescriptions. Any attempt to treat a medical condition should always come under the direction of a competent physician.

Acne

A lot of acne is the result of eating a diet high in sugar and low in fibre. When the body is not eliminating waste properly, the pores of the skin become blocked. It is very important to make sure that you eat plenty of vegetables that are rich in fibre (not wheat or wheat bran as in wholegrain bread as this tends to clog up people who suffer from acne and skin problems). Steer clear of processed convenience foods (they are full of the kind of hydrogenated fats you find in margarines) and stick to using olive oil for your salads and wok frying. Do a detox and use the High Life Diet, emphasizing the fresh vegetables and fruits. Avoid dairy products.

Carrot juice is very beneficial for acne, but the green juices are supreme. Drink lots and lots of fresh carrot juice, to which you add as much green as you can manage, as often as you can manage it. The best sources of green are cabbage and kale, beetroot and turnip tops, watercress and spinach, parsley and dandelion leaves.

Carrot & Apple *Ginger Spice*
Carrot High *Green Friend*
Chlorophyll Plus

Allergy

All allergies, from the classic antibody antigen reactions that cause the release of histamine, to food allergies which can act quite differently, must be treated holistically. That means diet, rest, stress management and the elimination of any possible trigger foods or environmental chemicals.

Sugar is the first thing that needs to be eliminated completely from the diet. Cut out packaged convenience foods that are full of additives such as aspartamine – the sulphites in prepared meat foods – and monosodium glutamate (MSG). Many allergic people have an overgrowth of candida albicans yeast in their bodies and need to address this at the same time. Milk products are best avoided by anyone with any sort of allergic condition.

Most allergic reactions occur when the body is overacidic. A high alkaline diet, such as a Raw Energy-type regime, plus lots of alfalfa sprouts or juice (which is rich in mineral salts) can help to create the right internal environment. Celery will also help you become allergy-free. Grapefruit, orange, cantaloupe and parsley are rich in the bioflavonoids; spinach, kale and sweet peppers are rich in B6, which can be particularly helpful for many sensitivities; garlic, spinach and cauliflower are a good source of molybdenum, a trace element that tends to be deficient in people who are sensitive to the sulphites and MSG.

Celery Sticks	*Red Cool*
Parsley Passion	*Sprout Special*

Anaemia

Anaemia occurs either when there is a decrease in the total number of red blood cells, or in the volume of the blood, or when red blood cells become abnormal in shape or size. This condition tends to make you pale and weak and inhibits your resistance to infection. It often creates insomnia, leading to irritability and depression and causing chronic fatigue. There are a number of different underlying deficiencies that are present when one is anaemic; iron is important in order to be able to form new red blood cells, and folic acid and vitamin B12 help to rebuild red blood cells. If anaemia persists, consult your doctor. It could possibly be the result of abnormalities in the production of haemoglobin itself.

Green drinks and green foods are essential for anaemia sufferers. They are rich in folic acid and many of them are rich in iron, particularly watercress, spinach, beetroot tops, dandelion leaves and the brassicas. Vegetables which are particularly beneficial include parsley, green pepper, beetroot tops, carrot, kale, spinach and asparagus. Berries can be very useful, particularly for women (they are good for menstrual cramps, morning sickness and calming labour pains, not to mention sea sickness, yeast infections and poor circulation).

Try to drink as many green drinks as possible. To each glass add a teaspoon of spirulina, which is extremely rich in B12, and shake or blend well.

Beet Treat	*Easy Does It*
Dandelion Plus	*Green Zinger*
Double Whammy	*Red Flag*

Arthritis

Both osteoarthritis and rheumatoid arthritis have been successfully treated with juice therapy, which is particularly beneficial if the patient has not been on long-term drug treatment. Osteoarthritis affects the bones and joints with symptoms such as swelling of soft tissues, local tenderness, restricted movement, bony swellings and crackings of the joints as well as stiffness after resting. The more the joint is used in osteoarthritis, the worse the pain generally becomes. Rheumatoid arthritis produces inflammatory conditions in the joints and the structures surrounding joints, as well as a feeling of weakness, often with low-grade fever, long-term fatigue, pain and stiffness. Rheumatoid arthritis is increasingly considered an auto-immune reaction where the body has actually developed antibodies against its own tissues.

In both osteo- and rheumatoid arthritis, certain things are essential. Firstly, that you cut out foods from the nightshade family such as potatoes, aubergine, tomatoes, and peppers. Secondly (in the case of osteoarthritis) that you avoid citrus fruits such as limes, lemons, oranges and grapefruits. In the tradition of natural medicine these are believed to contribute to the inflammation.

With both forms of arthritis, it is important to avoid all convenience foods and refined foods such as white sugar, white flour, processed foods that contain chemical additives, and alcohol. Consider the possibility that you might have some sort of a sensitivity or allergic reaction to food, perhaps to wheat or to dairy products. Try eliminating wheat flour and everything made from it as well as all dairy products from your diet for three weeks and see if it makes a significant difference. In the case of rheumatoid arthritis it can be useful, if you are not a vegetarian, to eat more cold water fish such as tuna, sardines, salmon and mackerel which contain the essential fatty acid known as omega-3. Many people with arthritis fare better on a low-fat vegetarian diet.

Vegetables to incorporate into your juices include carrot, beetroot tops, broccoli, turnip, grapes, kale, cabbage, all dark green vegetables, apple, and ginger. Pineapple is particularly good for rheumatoid arthritis since it contains the enzyme bromelin which has anti-inflammatory properties.

Dandelion juice is excellent, especially for rheumatoid arthritis. Pick the dandelion greens carefully, from places which are not likely to have been sprayed and are not along the verges of roads where they may have picked up heavy metals such as lead from air pollution. Cut off the leaves and wash them well before putting them through the juicer. If you are used to drinking green juices you can actually drink dandelion juice on its own, or mixed equally with carrot. It also mixes well with a little water-cress. If you are not used to drinking green juices, it can be useful to start with a delicious sweet juice such as carrot and apple and then gradually increase the levels of dandelion you are putting into it. Dandelion also has the ability to create an amazing high once the juice is assimilated into the liver, which usually takes about half an hour. But go easy, for if your digestive system is not used to green juices this can be too much of a shock. Start with small amounts and increase gradually.

Ginger Berry	*Popeye Punch*
Green Goddess	*Red Genius*
Green Wow	*Sprouting o' the Green*
Pineapple Green	*Top of the Beet*
Pineamint	

Asthma

The theory is that asthma comes in two forms. One kind is said to be caused by specific allergens either in the air or food; the other is said to have no particular cause. Most experts in natural medicine, however, find that there is always an allergic element, as there is also always an emotional one in any kind of asthma or other condition in which the symptoms include spasms of the bronchial tubes and swelling of the mucous membrane.

Perhaps the most important remedy is to eliminate from the diet any foods that create mucus in the body. This means not eating dairy products, coffee, tea, chocolate, wheat, and convenience foods. Many asthmatics find they do best when they eliminate from their diet not only wheat but other grains as well (except for buckwheat, which is not a true grain, and brown rice or millet). Asthmatics seem to be more affected by food allergies than other people, which can result in inflammation of the bronchial tubes that causes an even stronger reaction to smoke, pollen and air pollutants such as sulphur-dioxide. Asthma also appears to weaken the adrenal glands, so handling it means living on a low-allergy diet in which at least 50 per cent of the foods that you eat are taken raw.

Juices that are rich in magnesium, which relaxes the bronchial muscle, are particularly useful, including turnip, watercress, kale, turnip greens, parsley, collard greens, carrots, asparagus and beetroot tops. A couple of tablespoons of lemon juice added to any glass of fresh raw juice is a traditional treatment for asthma, as are molasses, which can be a useful additive to a glass of any juice. Other additives which are equally useful include fresh ginger, onions, and garlic (in small quantities, if you wish to keep your friends).

Carrot High	*Hi NRG*
Glorious Grapefruit	*Leslie's Cocktail*
Hi Mag	*Potassium Punch*

Cellulite

Orange peel skin – the lumps and bumps that are so hard to get rid of, even in slim women – can be shed provided you take a total body approach to the issue. Women with cellulite are often constipated, even if they have one bowel movement a day, and they also tend to have poor lymphatic drainage, so that wastes are not eliminated properly. In addition, many women with cellulite suffer from poor liver function and an under-active thyroid.

Foods that are rich in bioflavonoids such as sweet peppers, tomatoes, cabbage, parsley and citrus fruits (incorporate the pithy, white covering inside the peel in your juices) are important because they help strengthen the capillaries so you don't get leakage and the pockets of water that create *peau d'orange* flesh. Vitamin C is also important to strengthen the capillaries, as is zinc. If you want to shed cellulite permanently, shift the percentage of raw foods in your diet so that you are consuming between 50 and 75 per cent of your foods raw. Use skin brushing, cut out *all* convenience foods which are replete with junk fats and chemicals, and eliminate coffee and tea.

Remember that cellulite is slow to form and slow to clear, but it *will* go away provided you are persistent. These juices will be beneficial:

Ginger Berry	*Pineapple Green*
Ginger's Best	*Potassium Power*
Hi Mag	*Waterfall*

Colds

The common cold has for generations been considered by natural health practitioners to be the body's means of eliminating waste when it has become overloaded. When you feel yourself coming down with a cold eliminate all dairy products from your diet and all foods with sugar in them. Do a Juice Blitz and follow that by following the High Life Diet for at least a week.

Juicing for colds has two goals. The first is to strengthen the immune system, and for this you need lots of greens – kale, parsley, green pepper, watercress – which contain plenty of anti-oxidants such as beta-carotene (don't forget your carrots too) as well as vitamin C, chlorophyll and all of those as yet unexplained plant properties which are so strengthening to the body. The second purpose of juicing for colds is in many ways the most important and that is elimination. This means using juices from vegetables and fruits which help eliminate waste from the system. These include lemon, apricot, garlic, parsley, ginger, watercress, kale, radish, spinach, apple, pear and **tomato**.

Atomic Lift-Off	*Hi Mag*
Beetroot, Carrot &	*Pineapple Grapefruit Drink*
Orange	*Red Genius*
Carrot High	*Salad Juice*
Ginger Spice	*Sweet and Spicy*

Constipation

Constipation is the hidden condition that, according to natural health practitioners, is so widespread that it would be hard to quantify it. These experts insist that very few of us are actually cleansing our colon as thoroughly as we should. Most people find that when they begin to take juices and eat a higher percentage of their foods raw, their constipation clears by itself and they begin to have two or three bowel movements a day. It is essential to overall health that the bowels function really well, for if faecal matter stays in the colon then harmful substances from the natural bacteria that live in the bowel can contribute to the development of many specific ailments such as haemorrhoids, varicose veins, hernias, cellulite, flatulence, obesity, insomnia, bad breath, indigestion and diverticulitis. Constipation also plays a part in the development of degenerative diseases, from cancer to coronary heart disease, diabetes and even long-term depression.

One of the best natural remedies for constipation is rhubarb. Rhubarb is a vegetable but is usually thought of as a fruit. It is rich in calcium, phosphorus, iron, sodium, potassium, vitamin A, folic acid, vitamin C and magnesium. Raw rhubarb, like spinach, also contains oxalic acid, which you don't want to get too much of. Therefore rhubarb is not an ingredient we would use daily in any of our juices. Rhubarb is useful for intestinal parasites and for intestinal wind, and rhubarb juice applied externally is traditionally used to treat leg ulcers, bed sores and wounds. However, rhubarb juice and spinach juice should not be taken by anyone who suffers from kidney stones, because of their high oxalic acid content.

Getting over constipation is usually a simple matter once you begin to juice, but there are a number of juices that are especially useful during the transition stage. Rhubarb, apples, spinach, prunes and pears all have a natural laxative effect.

Apples & Pears	*Ginger's Best*
Beet Treat	*Rhubarb Radiance*
Black Watermelon	*Spinapple*
Carrot, Beet, Celery,	*Sprout Special*
Tomato	*Tropical Prune*

Depression

Feeling depressed is not just a psychological condition. Very often that sense of purposelessness, emptiness, feelings of worthlessness and guilt, come from a biochemical imbalance in the body. Internal pollution is a major cause, which is why a Juice Blitz plus a week on the High Life Diet shifts depression for many people.

Sugar and caffeine should be avoided and it is important to check for any food allergies. Nobody who is depressed should be eating convenience foods, even those so-called comfort foods that are supposed to cheer us up. The neurotransmitters – hormones in the brain which control feeling – are derived from the food we eat, so the food has got to be good. Serotonin (derived from the amino acid tryptophan) is a particularly significant neurotransmitter. When there are adequate levels of serotonin in the brain the mood tends to be elevated and sleep normal; low serotonin levels are associated with mood distortions and interrupted sleep patterns. A meal rich in complex carbohydrates helps the body absorb tryptophan, and therefore promotes the production of serotonin.

Bananas, figs and dates are rich in tryptophan. Carbohydrate in the form of a piece of toast and a banana before bed can help tremendously to induce sleep and also create a sense of calm peacefulness (provided, of course, that you are not allergic to the grains from which the toast is made).

To banish the blues permanently, increase the levels of raw food in your diet to between 50 and 75 per cent each day. Try using the Juice Blitz one day each week for a few weeks as well, to help continue the detoxification process. Meanwhile make your juices rich in dark green vegetables full of magnesium, potassium, iron, calcium and folic acid. A deficiency in any of these can contribute to depression, as can a deficiency in fatty acids, which is why it can be useful to add linseeds to your juices. Don't be discouraged if it takes a little time to deep-cleanse your body and replenish the nutrients you may be lacking. It is well worth the effort.

Chlorophyll Plus　　*Pineamint*
Ginger Spice　　*Red Genius*
Hi Mag　　*Salsa Surprise*
Linusit Perfect

Digestion

Digestive troubles come in many forms, from minor problems such as a bloated feeling after a meal, to abdominal pain and wind, nausea, and more serious ailments like gastric ulcers, diverticulitis, and colon troubles. In all these circumstances, it's important to avoid taking in any substances that can irritate the gut, such as coffee, alcohol and chocolate. Occasionally stomach troubles come from *hypochlorhydria* – a deficiency of hydrochloric acid – in which case pineapple and papaya juice are excellent since they are rich in the protein-digesting enzymes bromelin and papain.

Among clinical reports of juicing, none is more impressive than the results that Dr Garnett Cheney of Stanford University reported for his treatment of gastric ulcers using juices alone. Dr Cheney prescribed for his patients fresh raw green cabbage juice, prepared and drunk immediately. It contains anti-peptic ulcer factors which have a really quite remarkable effect.

Leslie's mother, who was diagnosed with a peptic ulcer at the age of 37 and who was very resistant to taking any form of medication, read about Cheney's work and began to use cabbage juice. She drank about five 300ml (8oz) glasses a day for six weeks and then took smaller quantities for several months. The ulcers cleared up and she was never troubled by them again.

Cabbage juice tends to benefit most digestive upsets. It's not exactly delicious, however, and it can be helpful to mix it with pineapple juice to soften the flavour. Ginger is also good for digestion and has been used for thousands of years to counteract nausea, travel sickness, and morning sickness. Bananas have been shown to help protect the stomach from excess hydrochloric acid. Most people with any digestive upset that is not a serious medical condition requiring treatment find that simply getting into a Juice High way of living clears up the problem. The following juices are especially good for that purpose:

Gingeroo	*Red Flag*
Ginger Spice	*Red Genius*
Pineappage	*Tropical Prune*

Eczema

An annoying condition that's often hard to get rid of, where the skin becomes red, swollen and itchy in the beginning, then later thickens to produce crusted, scaly patches, eczema has many causes. Allergies are often a prime factor, which makes it important to use an elimination diet and to check for any food allergies. With eczema, as with any skin condition, it is important that your elimination works properly so that your skin is not forced to eliminate waste the hard way. Try the Juice Blitz and the High Life Diet.

Certain nutrients are also very important in the treatment of eczema. Sweet peppers, tomatoes, cabbage and parsley are all excellent sources of bioflavonoids, which help reduce inflammation and control allergy, as well as enhancing the capillary function so you get a better flow of nutrients and elimination of waste from the skin. Citrus fruits are also good, provided you incorporate the pithy, white covering inside the peel in your juices. Zinc is particularly important. It's usually found in good quantities in carrots, garlic, parsley, and ginger. Carrot and parsley are also prime sources of beta-carotene as are kale and spinach.

Carrot & Apple	*Green Wow*
Chlorophyll Plus	*Parsley Passion*
Gingeroo	*Spring Salad*

Eye Health

The health of the eyes depends more than anything else on the quality of anti-oxidant protection that your body gets. Free radical damage is a major factor in the development of both minor eye problems, such as short-sightedness, to major problems, such as cataracts and glaucoma. For the eye to remain healthy it needs to be able to maintain a normal balance and concentration of such minerals as calcium, potassium and sodium within the lens. When free radical damage occurs the cellular mechanisms by which nutrients are pumped to the eyes and excess sodium and wastes removed no longer work so well. Beta-carotene, one of the most important of all of the bioflavonoids, is an anti-oxidant that helps protect the eye lens from ultra-violet damage.

Yellow, orange and dark green vegetables which are rich in beta-carotene as well as vitamins C and E, the B complex, zinc, calcium and phosphorus are very important for eye health. Ginger, garlic and parsley are rich in zinc, another mineral element that has been shown to be helpful. There is anecdotal evidence that drinking lots of carrot juice will improve eye sight, particularly night vision. Here are some of our favourite recipes for eyes.

Beet Treat	*Hi Mag*
Carrot & Apple	*Orange Tonic*
Double Whammy	*Pineapple Green*
Green Wild	*Spiked Celery*

Fatigue

One of the underlying causes of fatigue, particularly in women, can be iron depletion. Spinach juice is a far better way of boosting iron levels than taking tablets, which tend to be highly constipating and are not really absorbed very well. The iron in natural foods and juices such as spinach, or any of the green leafy vegetables, and also in legumes, poultry, whole grains, liver and molasses, is highly bioavailable, i.e. your body has no trouble making use of it. Remember that replenishing the body with essential nutrients takes time and so be prepared to work with natural foods and juices for several weeks before you start to see lasting relief from chronic fatigue.

Again, make sure that 50–75 per cent of the foods you eat each day are raw and make sure you get lots of chlorophyll-rich foods. Cereal grasses are good, as they are high in minerals, vitamins and enzymes and also have a wonderful ability to enliven the liver and thereby to create more energy. Chlorophyll also helps protect from infectious diseases. You can take wheat and barley-grass juice as a supplement in powdered form that you add to your vegetables and fruit juices or you can go the whole hog and get a cereal grass juicer and grow your own cereal grasses (see Resources, p. 436).

Magnesium is another important mineral when it comes to fatigue. Low intracellular magnesium makes the body very prone to infection, food allergies and chronic conditions. Good sources of magnesium are any of the dark green vegetables, whole grains, seaweeds, molasses, legumes, fish and nuts.

Atomic Lift-Off	*Hi Mag*
Citrusucculent	*Hit the Grass*
Dandelion Plus	*Parsley Passion*
Ginger Berry	*Secret of the Sea*
Gingeroo	*Spinapple*
Glorious Grapefruit	*Sprout Special*
Green Zinger	

Hair Loss

You may be genetically programmed to lose your hair, but that doesn't mean you have to let it go easily. There is a great deal you can do to prevent hair loss and at the very least slow it down dramatically. Eat more foods that are rich in sulphur, amino acids, L-methionine and L-cysteine. Eggs are good, but cabbage is king.

Sugars will tend to increase the rate of hair loss so try to eliminate sugar completely from your diet. Include in your diet plenty of foods which are rich in PABA, inositol and choline, such as mushrooms, spinach, legumes, lentils, brown rice. Consider adding a supplement of vacuum-packed flaxseeds to your diet. You can grind them in a coffee grinder and sprinkle them on salads or cereals in the morning. You can also add them to your juices.

Finally, the grain alfalfa, particularly in its sprouted form, has long been believed to stimulate hair growth. Other juices for incipient slapheads include:

Alfalfa – Father of all Juices

Carrot High

Fatty Acid Frolic

Ginger's Best

Parsnip Perfect

Spinapple

Hangover

The inevitable consequence of over-indulgence is waking up feeling dehydrated and nauseous, with a brain that feels as if it's banging against the side of your head when you move. You need to replenish your bodily fluids, renutrify exhausted muscles and get your head together. Fruit juice is strongly indicated. Citrus juices, being full of natural sugar and vitamin C, are the most immediately effective remedy, but they may be a bit harsh if your stomach is delicate. Watermelon, being exceptionally mild, is ideal.

There is an art to hangover management and the key to it is regarding detoxification as the corollary of intoxication. All drugs provoke a strongly acidic reaction in the body which causes the symptoms of a hangover and the first step to recovery is to correct the body's chemical imbalance. Plain old Carrot & Apple juice is effective for re-balancing and it's easy to take when you're feeling weak. Beet juice will greatly assist the repair of any possible damage done to your liver and kidneys.

Apples & Pears

Beet Treat

Carrot & Apple

Merry Belon

Virgin Mary

Insomnia

Insomnia can have many causes. Drugs such as beta blockers or thyroid medication, even caffeine and alcohol can all disrupt sleep. So, ironically, can sleeping pills, if your body becomes addicted to them.

Getting regular exercise – taking long walks rather than going to aerobics classes and throwing your back out of place – can help enormously to reduce the nervous tension that prevents sleep. Sometimes sleep is disrupted by hypoglycaemia, so make sure you don't have a blood sugar problem (see *Low Blood Sugar* below). Eliminate coffee, tea, alcohol and junk foods – including diet colas – from your life once and for all. Eat your biggest meal at lunchtime, as everyone sleeps better (and longer) when their stomach is not full. Consider using one of the well-proven natural tranquillisers such as Valerian, Passiflora (Passion flower) or Wild Lettuce. You can make a night-cap cocktail to help increase the levels of serotonin in the brain: blend a pinch of one of these natural tranquillisers into it.

Magnesium, vitamin B6 and niacin have to be present in order for the amino acid tryptophan to be able to turn itself into serotonin. Carrots are a rich source of all three. Calcium induces muscle relaxation and so does folic acid which in sufficient quantities prevents leg twitching and calms nervous tension. The green drinks, from dandelion to parsley and spinach, are excellent sources of folic acid and calcium. Seaweed is also a good source of magnesium. Many people (except those with low blood sugar) need an extra boost of fruit sugar before going to bed to trigger sleep. Pineapple and grape is a wonderful combination for this. Others include:

Green Goddess	*Smooth as Silk*
Hi Mag	*Spicy Carrot*
Lazy Lettuce	*Sprout Special*
Pineamint	

Low Blood Sugar (Hypoglycaemia)

Low blood sugar, where the body tends to secrete insulin which in turn makes the blood sugar level drop depriving the brain of its main 'food', glucose, is a condition that underlies much of the chocolate munching and coffee drinking that people indulge in in order to keep themselves going.

Hypoglycaemia involves disturbance to the balance of hormones in the body and can produce an enormous number of periodic symptoms including palpitations of the heart, sweating, depression, anxiety, headaches, poor concentration and bad temper. These symptoms are alleviated by munching on some sort of carbohydrate, such as a slice of wholegrain bread. The trick in clearing up the condition, however, is to clear out of your life everything that would trigger the pancreas to over-secrete insulin. In particular this means no sugar, chocolate, or bottled fruit juices. Choose foods that are rich in complex carbohydrates and fibre such as raw vegetables, whole oats, beans, wholegrain pasta, lentils, chick peas, etc. Sprouted seeds are particularly useful.

The vegetable juices are better than the fruit juices until blood sugar is stabilized. If you're hypoglycaemic, don't drink fruit juices unless they are well diluted with mineral water, and then only a couple of times a week. Try adding a little turmeric or cinnamon to your juices. Both these spices have long been used to help stabilize blood sugar. Foods which are rich in chromium will help regulate glucose metabolism in the body. These include spinach, apples, green peppers, whole grains, clams and liver. Use foods which are rich in manganese such as carrots, celery, beetroot, beetroot greens, turnip greens, pineapple, liver, eggs, green vegetables and buckwheat.

An antidote for a sweet tooth is lots of green drinks,

but you will have to get yourself used to drinking them since they are about the last thing the hypoglycaemic wants. Once you do get used to it you will find that blood sugar stabilizes and you have energy to spare, day in and day out. All of the green juices are excellent, such as:

Dandelion Plus	*Parsley Passion*
Green Friend	*Secret of the Sea*
Green Zinger	*Spicy Apple*
Lemon Zinger	*Tossled Carrot*

Migraine

When Leslie was 25 years old, she met a doctor who taught her about supporting the body to heal itself using juices and raw foods. Dr Philip Kilsby experienced 99 per cent success in the treatment of migraine, using juices, lots of raw fruits and vegetables, and a few dietary supplements. The only case of migraine he had not been able to cure was that of a woman who turned out not to have migraine but a brain tumour.

Kilsby taught that all migraine, regardless of cause, is centred in a liver that is over-worked trying to keep the body internally clear. So Kilsby took stress off the liver by removing from the diet foods that people are commonly allergic to such as red wine, other alcohol, salad cream, red plums, soft cheeses, figs, aged game, chicken liver, canned meat, salami sausages, pickled herring, aubergine, soy sauce and yeast concentrates, as well as chocolate, wheat, milk, the food colouring tartrazine, sugar, coffee and peanuts.

Kilsby then put his patients on a detox programme very much like the Juice Blitz, and followed it with a regime similar to the High Life Diet. Kilsby insisted his patients drink a juice rich in green vegetables twice daily. He found that his patients experienced migraines of decreasing intensity until, once their bodies were detoxified, the migraines altogether ceased.

Migraines result from contraction followed by rapid dilatation of the blood vessels in the brain, and this can be triggered by certain foods. Biofeedback can be helpful: this involves training yourself to visualize your hands as warm, thereby drawing blood away from the head and taking pressure off the area that is involved in the migraine. The herb feverfew can also be useful to many people.

If you suffer from migraine banish all chemicals, including artificial sweeteners such as aspartamine, from your diet. Include in your juices some of the fruits and vegetables which are known to reduce platelet stickiness, since foods that inhibit blood clotting are known to reduce migraine. These include garlic, cantaloupe, and ginger.

Dandelion Plus	*Green Goddess*
Gingeroo	*Spring Salad*
Green Friend	*Sprout Special*

Prostate Trouble

Enlargement of the prostate is so common that 60 per cent of men between the ages of 40 and 59 have the condition, which is properly known as benign prostatic hyperplasia (BPH). When this occurs there is an obstruction of the bladder outlet, increased frequency of urination and difficulty in urinating. The standard medical treatment for BPH is surgery. However, there is a great deal that can be done to improve the condition through nutrition. BPH is a hormone-dependent disorder of the metabolism. Testosterone, especially free testosterone levels, decrease after the age of 55. Meanwhile levels of other hormones increase, particularly those of a very potent male hormone called dihydrotestosterone within the prostate itself which is responsible for the over-production of prostate cells. This ultimately results in the enlarged prostate.

Protecting yourself against high levels of xenoestrogens from the environment is an important part of diminishing prostate enlargement. You should also aim to reduce your stress levels, and to eliminate beer from your diet. The mineral zinc and vitamin B6 have been shown to have a beneficial effect: zinc, in particular, has been shown to reduce the size of the prostate and to reduce symptoms in men who suffer from BPH. Similarly, essential fatty acids such as those found in organic linseed or flaxseed oil have been shown to bring about a significant improvement in many patients with the condition.

It is important that sufferers from prostate trouble are protected as much as possible from pesticides, herbicides and other petrochemically derived compounds in the environment such as biphenyls, hexachlorobenzene and dioxin, which can increase the formation of dihydrotestosterone in the prostate. Go for juices that are high in zinc and B6 and drinks containing organically grown, vacuum-packed linseeds or flaxseeds.

Dandelion Plus	*Green Zinger*
Ginger's Best	*Linusit Perfect*
Ginger Spice	*Pineapple Green*
Green Friend	*Silky Strawberries*

Pre-Menstrual Syndrome

PMS comes in many forms and causes many symptoms, from irritability, depression, tension and decreased energy, to backache, breast pain, changes in libido, abdominal bloating, oedema and headache. There are certain things that all PMS sufferers need to watch. It is essential to clear sugar out of your diet as well as cut down on any other form of refined carbohydrates, including white flour and honey. Avoid coffee, tea and chocolate, for two reasons – first because they contain *methylxanthines*, which have been linked with a number of the symptoms associated with PMS, and secondly, because anything containing caffeine can have a very negative effect on such things as breast tenderness, anxiety and depression.

It is also a good idea to eliminate all milk products and wheat from your diet for seven days prior to menstruation. At the same time increase your intake of certain nutrients such as magnesium, B6 and the B complex, as well as beta-carotene. Bromelin too can be helpful since this enzyme is believed to help relax the smooth muscle tissue of the body. Go for the green juices, which are rich in all these things. If you have water retention, turn towards watermelon, grape, cucumber and dandelion, each of which has a splendid ability to eliminate excess water from the system. You are likely to find that all the juices that are good for PMS are also useful for someone who is wrestling with menopausal symptoms such as hot flushes. In both PMS and menopausal cases it can be helpful to follow a Raw Energy way of eating where 50–75 per cent of your foods are taken raw during the 7–10 days before a period or whenever the symptoms seem to be at their worst.

Black Watermelon	*Pineapple Special*
Cool as a Cuke	*Secret of the Sea*
Ginger Berry	*Spring Salad*
Green Zinger	*Sprout Special*
Hi Mag	*Waterfall*
Pineapple Green	

Stress

Stress is a complicated condition to treat as it has many causes and takes many forms. However, whenever the body is under prolonged stress the tissues tend to become more acidic. There is nothing better and more life-changing that you can do when your system is too acid than to drink fresh vegetable and fruit juices to alkalinise it. Detoxification helps eliminate the constant tension, anxiety and frustration that so often go with stress, as well its common consequences such as gastro-intestinal difficulties, high blood pressure, dizziness, loss of appetite or excessive appetite, and headaches.

While it is important to practise some sort of deep relaxation or meditation if you are suffering from prolonged stress, the effect of dietary change alone, incorporating a juice-high regime into your lifestyle and as always making between 50 and 75 per cent of your foods raw can literally transform your life within a fortnight. Useful nutrients include pantothenic acid, which occurs in good quantity in green leafy vegetables such as kale, dandelion and broccoli; potassium, which is found in bananas, parsley and spinach; zinc, a good source of which are carrots and ginger; and magnesium, which also occurs in the green foods.

Easy Does It	*Hi Mag*
Gingeroo	*Hit the Grass*
Ginger Spice	*Silky Strawberries*
Green Friend	*Sprout Special*

Urinary Infections

Cranberry juice is excellent for any sort of kidney and urinary infections. Cranberry is also thought to be good for an under-active thyroid, partly because it has traditionally been grown, particularly in the United States, in iodine-rich bogs. Cranberry juice on its own is much too strong for most people to handle. However, it mixes beautifully with any number of gentler juices like melon or apple. It will also add extra zest to basic vegetable juices like carrot. Cranberry is known for its cleansing properties, helping to rid not only the digestive system but other organs of the body of waste and bacteria. It is also said to be very good for skin problems such as acne.

Cranberry Cocktail

Water Retention

Water retention or oedema is a sign that the metabolism is not working properly and the body needs to be deep cleansed and rebalanced. It can be caused by many things, from hormones in birth control pills and Hormone Replacement Therapy, to hormone changes during the premenstruum and pregnancy. It can also be caused by food allergies and liver problems.

Encouraging the body to eliminate excess water from its tissues is a two-fold process. First, use natural diuretics such as nettle, dill, watermelon, grapes and cucumber that gently encourage the loss of excess water. Second, detoxify the system as a whole using the Juice Blitz. If swelling in the ankles is severe and prolonged it can indicate serious problems such as heart failure, so you need to check with your doctor. Check also for any possibility of food allergy if you have prolonged water retention, and decrease the amount of salt in your diet. The sodium/potassium balance in your body determines to a great extent whether the body eliminates excess fluids properly. Cut sugar from your diet.

Fight water retention by increasing the number of potassium-rich foods that you eat and make your juices from. These include: bananas, prunes, raisins, figs, seaweeds, fish, green vegetables, whole grains, kale, broccoli, spinach, Swiss chard, and all the other green foods, plus carrot and celery. You may be deficient in vitamin B6, which can interfere with the kidneys' ability to eliminate waste. Foods rich in B6 include molasses, brown rice, liver, eggs, cabbage and fish. Garlic, too, is one of the traditional foods for eliminating oedema from the tissues.

Black Watermelon	*Green Zinger*
Cool as a Cuke	*Potassium Power*
Dandelion Plus	*Secret of the Sea*
Green Friend	

7
Green Lightning

Once you get the basics of juicing under your belt – once you get used to the wild raw taste of fresh vegetables – you are ready for the next step: *green lightning*. And what a step it is. Green juices, like the foods they are pressed from, are little short of magical. They bring you increased energy, protection from radiation in the environment and from degenerative diseases as well as enhanced immune performance. Green foods help regenerate and rejuvenate the body. Go green and you can wave those annoying winter colds and 'flu good bye. The old adage 'eat your greens if you want to stay young and healthy' is now scientific fact. And the fun of it all is that, so far, advanced nutritional scientists know that green works wonders but nobody is yet sure why. The chlorophyll? The enzymes? Mystery ingredients? The very latest nutritional supplements have gone green – spirulina, chlorella, green barley, blue-green algae. The nutrients they contain – from vitamins and minerals to trace elements, enzymes and as yet unidentified health-promoting factors – are found there in perfect balance and synergy as well as in a highly bioavailable form. Your system just laps them up.

Bountiful Brassicas

Dark green vegetables such as broccoli, Brussels sprouts, collards, kale, kohlrabi and mustard greens have hit the headlines in the last few years thanks to an overwhelming abundance of medical and scientific evidence that they

271

help prevent cancer. Prestigious North American medical journals such as the *Journal of the National Cancer Institute* and *Federation Proceedings* report that the sulphur and histidine in brassicas inhibit the growth of cancer tumours, detoxify the system of poisonous environmental chemicals, prevent colon cancer and increase the body's own supply of natural cancer-fighting compounds. They can also help lower low-density lipoproteins – the *bad* cholesterol – which accompany hardening of the arteries. They improve elimination and fight yeast infections too. Adding a couple of florets of broccoli or a few leaves of kale to a glass of carrot juice turns something good into something even better. But start slowly and gradually build up on the green. In the beginning – especially if you have a sweet tooth or if you are addicted to sugar – the taste can seem pretty strong. Build up gradually until you find that your old craving for sugars has actually been transformed into a new craving for green.

Grass That's Greener

Another group of green lightning foods, the cereal grasses, are some of the least known but most powerful green foods. You need special equipment to extract the juice from them, but these grasses are also sold in health food shops as a dried powder and can be stirred into raw juice by the teaspoonful. Of course grasses have been around for thousands of years, yet only in the last ten or fifteen years has the consumption of young grass – wheat or rye or oat or barley – begun to rise. In ancient times young cereal plants were treated with the respect they deserve. Tiny green tips of baby wheat plants were eaten as a delicacy in the Holy Land 2,000 years ago. Then in the twenties and thirties, in the United States – before vitamin and mineral pills were in existence – bottled, dehydrated cereal grass became a popular food supplement.

Young grasses are very different from the mature grains they eventually turn into from which we make our breads and porridge. Dark green in colour, in some ways they are similar to dark green brassica vegetables in their protective abilities. But they are very special. When rice, wheat, corn, oats, barley, rye or millet are planted in good healthy soil with plenty of rainfall and are harvested at exactly the right moment not only do they taste sweet, but are unbelievably rich in vitamins and minerals, enzymes and growth hormones you would be hard pressed to find elsewhere. They are *living foods* and the juice pressed from them carries these life energies into your body. The young germinated plant is a little miracle of nature. In the young leaves photosynthesis produces simple sugars which are transformed into proteins, fatty acids, nucleic acids such as DNA and RNA as well as complex carbohydrates through the action of enzymes and substrates produced from minerals in the soil. The peak of nutritional bounty in all cereal grasses – the moment when chlorophyll, protein and most of the vitamins and minerals reach their zenith – occurs just before *jointing*. This is the moment at which the young internodal tissue in the grass leaf starts to elongate and form a stem. This is when cereal grasses are best harvested – usually somewhere between 8 and 15 days after planting. Afterwards the chlorophyll, protein and vitamin content drops dramatically while the fibre content increases rapidly. To give you some idea of just how remarkable the nutritional content of young cereal grasses can be it is useful to compare fresh wheat grass to freshly milled wholewheat flour:

Nutrients per 100 grammes dry weight:

	Wheat Grass	Wholewheat Flour
Chlorophyll (mg)	543	0
Vitamin A (iu)	23,136	0
Total Dietary Fibre (gm)	37	10
Protein (gm)	32	13
Carbohydrates (gm)	37	71
Calcium (mg)	277	41
Vitamin C	51	0
Iron	34	4
Folic Acid (mcg)	100	38
Niacin (mg)	6.1	4.3
Riboflavin (mg)	2.03	0.12

Green Blood

In 1928 the American chemist Charles Schnabel was searching for some material that could be added to poultry feeds to improve egg production and lower chicken mortality. He wanted what he described as a 'blood building material'. Scientists had discovered that chlorophyll – the green substance in plants – has a remarkable similarity in its chemical structure to haemoglobin – the oxygen-carrying element in animal blood. Schnabel figured that 'green leaves should be the best source of blood.' So he began to feed all sorts of green things to chickens – from alfalfa to combinations of twenty green vegetables. But he found them all wanting. Then he tried giving hens a green mixture which 'just happened to contain a large amount of immature wheat and oats.' Animals who got only 10 per cent of this cereal grass responded amazingly. Winter egg production shot up from an average of 38 per cent to 94 per cent of summer levels and the eggs that were produced had stronger shells and hatched healthier chicks.

Intrigued by his success with chickens, Schnabel began to investigate every aspect of cereal grasses – from the soils that produce the most nutritionally rich grasses to the effect that giving dehydrated grasses has on the health of humans. He also fed his own family of seven on them and was known to boast that none of them ever had a serious illness or a decayed tooth. He even developed a vision of how to feed the hungry of the world on the exceedingly high quality protein from cereal grasses.

The Grass Juice Factor

In the decades that followed other scientists working with animal nutrition confirmed that a mixture of young cereal grasses fed to livestock improved milk production in cows and produced stronger more resilient, longer-living animals – from guinea pigs and rats to rabbits, cats and ferrets. Others discovered that green cereal grass feeds, which are believed to contain natural plant steroid hormones, both enhanced fertility and improved lactation in many animals including humans. Since then scientists have done their best to isolate and identify the ingredient or ingredients in young cereal grasses responsible for all of this. Further research indicates that barley grass juice lowers serum cholesterol and that wheat grass, in addition to its rejuvenating powers, may have anti-cancer properties.

Those in the know have been making practical use of grasses for many years. Ann Wigmore, the founder of the Hippocrates Health Institute in Boston, has long promoted the use of wheat grass and wheat grass juice as well as green and raw foods in the treatment of chronic degenerative conditions.

Quantum Sunlight

Chlorophyll – the stuff that makes plants green – is an important health-promoting ingredient in young cereal grasses and green foods. The chlorophyll molecule has an ability to convert the energy of the sun into chemical energy through the mysterious process of photosynthesis. It is the chlorophyll molecule that enables plants to make carbohydrates out of carbon dioxide and water. All life on earth draws its power to be from the sun's energy, thanks to photosynthesis in plants.

Scientists now tend to believe that the remarkable health-promoting qualities of green plants reside in the synergistic effect of chlorophyll together with other vital nutrients, both known and unknown, that are found in the plants. H.E. Kirchner, who spent many years investigating the power of cereal grasses and green foods, has written, 'Chlorophyll, the healer, is at once powerful and bland – devastating to germs, yet gentle to wounded body tissues. Exactly how it works is still Nature's secret; to the layman, at least, the phenomenon seems like green magic.' Little wonder that for thousands of years the leaves and green stems of plants have been used for supporting detoxification of the body, wound healing, deodorisation, and any number of other purposes.

Chlorophyll is known to inhibit the carcinogenic effects of exposure to simple environmental poisons such as coal dust and tobacco, and to foods such as red wine and fried beef. In fact chlorophyll used on its own for these purposes has been proved to be more effective than the anti-oxidant vitamins A, C and E. Simple chlorophyll also helps protect from radiation. And when two or more of the dark green vegetables and cereal grasses are used together an animal's resistance to radiation reaches a peak. Chlorophyll also inhibits the growth of bacteria by creating an environment in which they simply do not reproduce. It also decreases swelling and reduces inflammation and speeds wound healing while reducing itching, irritation and pain. The chlorophyll-rich green juices come into their own in the treatment of peptic ulcers and are also useful in the relief of a range of conditions including constipation, spastic colitis and halitosis.

Ask Any Weed

Some of the very best of the green foods to add to your raw energy juices are weeds – plants that grow wild in your garden or in fields and hedgerows in the country. Dandelions, nettles, ragweed and Lamb's Quarter are especially good sources of the minerals and trace elements that we tend to lack as a result of chemical farming. Nettles, for example, only grow on mineral-rich soils. A handful of young nettles (they don't sting yet) gives a great boost to a glass of carrot and apple juice. Dandelion, like nettle, is a natural diuretic – which is why in French its common name is *pissenlit* – and a blood cleanser and is stunningly rich in the carotenoids. Lamb's Quarter is not only rich in minerals but also tastes delicious and can be used in salads as well as juices without imparting too heavy a green flavour to whatever you are making. Comfrey, in small quantities, can be added to fresh juice. It is rich in allantoin which herbalists have long used to soothe intestinal irritations such as stomach ulcers and diarrhoea as well as to calm skin eruptions and heal wounds.

Seaweeds too are great additives to juicing. You can use powdered kelp, dried nori, arame, hiziki, laver bread, dulse, kombu and wakami or you can even slip a piece of fresh seaweed taken from unpolluted waters in the juicer next to your carrot. Seaweeds are full of trace elements which are essential to the body in minute quantities – elements such as boron, chromium, cobalt, calcium, iodine, magnesium, manganese, molybdenum, phosphorus, potassium, silicon and sulphur. Unlike the chalk which is added to bread to 'enrich' it with calcium, and most of the mineral supplements you buy in pill form in stores, the minerals in green plants such as these are *organic* which means that your body can easily make use of them to build health.

The Ultra Greens

Watercress and parsley are superb additions to your juices. They are ultra green and very powerful so you need very little to get a lot of benefit from them. Watercress contains many more organic minerals than spinach and is richer in vitamins too. It has a high sulphur content which experts in natural medicine claim helps to improve the functioning of the endocrine system. Thanks to its iron, manganese and copper content, it is also known to be good for strengthening the blood and relieving anaemia. And it is rich in vitamins C and E. Parsley is another natural diuretic – great for cleansing the body of wastes and reducing oedema. It is famous for its ability to improve the health of the kidneys and for its anti-oxidant compounds including beta-carotene. Like watercress juice, parsley juice is super-potent both in taste and in actions – you need only a stalk or two of either plant to turn any juice you are making into a green powerhouse.

Good, Better, Best

You can go green in three ways. Firstly, you can add a handful – a small one at first until you get used to green juicing – of kale or broccoli or dark green cabbage to a simple base such as half carrot and half apple. Secondly – and better still – you can grow organic cereal grasses like wheat grass or barley in trays and harvest as you need them (but you will need special equipment to juice them, as described in Resources, p. 432) to add to your vegetable juices. Finally, you can buy freeze-dried wheat grass or green barley or one of the other green magic foods such as spirulina or chlorella and add them to whatever juice you fancy.

Magic Spirals

Use the nutritious natural green additives freely. They will do you nothing but good. Queen of them all is spirulina. A near-microscopic, blue-green freshwater alga, spirulina is one of the finest green additives you will ever find. It is made up of translucent bubble-thin cells stacked end to end to form an incredibly beautiful green helix. 3½ billion years ago the blue-green algae began to fix nitrogen from the atmosphere and to convert it into carbon dioxide and sugars, releasing free oxygen in the process. This created the oxygen-rich atmosphere in which the rest of life was able to develop.

Spirulina is probably the single most important nutritional supplement you can use to support high-level health. It is unusual in that its protein is alkaline forming in the body rather than acid-forming. This can be very important for detoxifying the system and also for helping you deal with high levels of stress. Spirulina is also rich in vitamins E, B12, C, B1, B5 and B6 as well as beta-carotene, and the minerals zinc, copper, manganese and selenium. It also contains good levels of anti-ageing anti-oxidants and of *phycocyanin* – a blue pigment structurally similar to beta-carotene which experiments have shown can enhance immune functions. Finally, spirulina although very low in fat is rich in important essential fatty acids. Add between a teaspoon and a tablespoon to a glass of fresh juice, or mix a glass of fresh juice together with spirulina and a banana in a blender for a great breakfast drink.

Emerald Treasure

Chlorella, sometimes called the emerald food, is a green alga with pretty amazing properties, and it too is great as a juice additive. It gets its name from its high content of chlorophyll – the highest of any known plant. In addition it is rich in vitamins, minerals, fibre, nucleic acids, amino acids, enzymes, something called CGF – chlorella growth factor – and other important compounds. Chlorella is the biggest-selling health food supplement in Japan. Among the green foods, chlorella is known as the great normaliser, thanks to its apparent ability to alter bodily processes that are under- or over-active so that they return to normal. About 60 per cent of chlorella is protein. The vitamins it contains include vitamin C, beta-carotene and other carotinoids, thiamin, riboflavin, pyridoxine, niacin, pantothenic acid, folic acid, vitamin B12, biotin, choline, vitamin K, inositol and PABA. Chlorella is also rich in minerals and trace elements including phosphorus, potassium, magnesium, sulphur, iron, calcium, manganese, copper, zinc and cobalt.

Japanese scientists have discovered that chlorella can stimulate the production of white blood cells and enhance immunity as well as having anti-viral activity. It can also bind heavy metals such as cadmium, pesticide and herbicide poisons including PCB, and help remove them from the body. Meanwhile it helps protect the liver from toxic injury, and some practitioners claim it can help prevent hangovers by promoting the removal of alcohol from the body.

Easy Does It

The secret with using any of the green lightning foods – from crunchy broccoli to wheat grass or spirulina – is to start small and keep adding as you get used to the green. Generally speaking the worse your diet has been before you begin the less you will like the taste of the green foods at first. This is particularly true if you have always been a big sugar eater. Green lightning and sugar are at the opposite ends of the food continuum. This may be one of the reasons why going green with your juices is about the best thing you can do to counter low blood sugar, low energy problems or candida albicans. But once you get used to green you will love not only the way it makes you feel and look but even the way it tastes – so fresh and clean and alive.

Quantum Green Drink

Many green foods have strong plant structures and therefore can be difficult to break down in a juicer. That is why we prefer, when using watercress or parsley or one of the weeds, to pulverize them quickly in the blender by themselves before adding a freshly made glass of raw carrot, celery or apple juice and whisking the mixture together for a few seconds. This way you produce a therapeutic green drink that is equal to none. We have learned much from H.E. Kirchner, a world authority on the benefits of green foods. Here is our version of his famous 'Green Drink'. We call it Quantum Green.

Make a glass of carrot and apple juice or fresh pineapple juice. Pour it into a blender and add a handful of sunflower seeds (which have been soaked in spring water overnight) as well as half the quantity of almonds and five dates without their stones. Now put in a handful or two of green leaves or sprouted green foods such as alfalfa or mung beans. Choose from comfrey, Lamb's Quarter, dandelion, parsley, mint, watercress, kale or beet top – using the leaves only, never the stems. Now liquefy the greens by blending for a few moments.

This is a rich protein food and an ideal meal replacement. If you want a less high-protein drink, leave out the seeds and nuts or cut their quantities in half.

Experiment with the green recipes on pages 297–9 and see what you come up with for yourself. Then let us know. We are always eager to find new ways of playing with green lightning.

8

Juice Freedom

We have examined the biochemical effect living juices have on the body. We have looked at the practicality of juicing and all the rites and rituals of deep cleansing and energizing the body. But what can you expect from carrying out a Juice Blitz and then following the High Life Diet? What is it going to do for you? What are the real payoffs?

The Bottom Line

There are many, many rewards to be gleaned from the Juice High lifestyle. Your body gets healthier, energy soars, skin is clearer and less lined, eyes are brighter, weight problems lessen, and chronic depression or anxiety start to become things of the past. However, the truth is that when it comes to regular juicing and a Raw Energy lifestyle, nothing less than *freedom* is the bottom line. Incorporating the power of Raw Energy day after day into your life can not only bring freedom *from* negative experiences such as chronic fatigue and illness by strengthening immunity and deep cleansing of the body. It can also bring you freedom *to* do things – to be more creative and live out what you really are. Deep cleansing and regeneration help set people free. For we live in a difficult time, one which demands focused awareness and knowledge if we are to handle not only the physical toxicity in our environment but also the spiritual and emotional toxicity that distort our perceptions and limit the full expression of the unique soul energy which is within each one of us.

Only you can prove this for yourself by moving beyond

theory and getting into your own juicing programme. Then you can experience for yourself just how wonderful a personal revolution it can bring about.

Expand Your Horizons

When you detox your body you remove impediments to experience and to action. You release energy that has been suppressed beneath the physical burden of waste which we all carry. But the energy which is released needs to be channelled. While for most people the increase in energy which comes with a Juice High lifestyle grows gradually and steadily, for some it can be experienced as an explosion of life force which suddenly arises from within. This was Leslie's experience the first time she ever did a juice fast. This is her story:

'I had an important decision to make about my life, and I felt that I had neither the clarity nor the information I needed in order to be able to make it wisely. A doctor friend of mine who was an expert in detoxification suggested I try a fast. At first this sounded completely insane to me. What possible bearing could drinking juices and water have on decision making? Then he told me about all the ancient practices of using fasting for intellectual and spiritual ends. I learned how monks and nuns were fasted to clarify their inner vision and bring them spiritual awareness, how Pythagoras fasted for forty days and then insisted that his students fast also before sitting exams, and that the famous Swiss physician Paracelsus insisted that "Of all the remedies available, fasting is the greatest one." And I began to wonder.'

Gateway To Power

The Juice Blitz is but a milder form of detoxification than a fast on spring water. It will do the same thing but more slowly and more gently. And it is much easier on your system. It also has the advantage of not depleting your body of minerals and trace elements, as well as vitamins and other as yet unidentified metabolites which are central to high level health. The High Life Diet will continue the detoxification processes – yet more slowly and more gently still – while it carries through the metabolic building process to help restore first-rate biochemical functioning on which high-level health, emotional balance and mental and spiritual clarity depend.

'Still not entirely convinced, I began my juice fast which I continued for 21 days under medical supervision. (This is the only way in which such a long juice fast should be carried out. More than two or three days on juice alone needs careful monitoring by a professional who understands and has experience with detoxification.) The results of my juicing quite literally changed my life. As a child and while I was growing up I had suffered endless illness – colds, flu, high fevers and nightmares every night. Then in my early twenties I found myself imprisoned by a heavy, long-term depression with no apparent cause for which no professional – doctor, psychologist or counsellor – could find a cure. Unknown to me it was juicing that would hold the key.

In the first five days on juice I experienced the odd headache and a great deal of fatigue since my body was throwing off waste at a fantastic rate. This temporarily depleted my energy for action so I rested as much as I could. Then the whole world began to look different. My body felt light instead of the burden I had for years experienced it to be. My eyes grew bright. But what amazed me most of all was that my whole experience of who I was began to shift. So did the way I viewed myself, my life, and the world around me.

Before my juice fast I had experienced myself as someone struggling against great odds day by day to just to raise my children and find my place in the world. During the detox I noticed that my image of myself and my attitudes towards life were undergoing subtle yet profound shifts. I began to see clearly and to feel that with steady commitment and patience I could accomplish what I wanted with my children and my work. I found that each day I would wake up free of the old anxieties, feeling fresh and excited about the day ahead.'

Wonderful Life

Someone once told Leslie a story about a psychologist who was studying the nature of optimism and pessimism in children. It's a story about just how different the world can look – depending on your attitude to life.

The psychologist filled a room with a tremendous array of toys of the kind that appeal to an eight-year-old – trains and trucks, building materials, stuffed toys, story books, painting and drawing materials. Then he took an eight-year-old *pessimist* and put him in the room while he and the child's mother waited in an adjoining office to see how long the child would amuse himself. In less than ten minutes the child came out of the room whining, 'Mummy, I'm bored. There's nothing to do in there.'

Next the psychologist replaced everything in the room with a large pile of horse manure. This time he sent an eight-year-old *optimist* into the room and closed the door, expecting that at any moment child would emerge. Instead, silence. Ten minutes passed. Then twenty. Finally an hour went by with no sign of the child. The child's mother voiced concern that perhaps her son had hurt himself. The psychologist let her open the door to see if her son was all right. Hearing the door open, the boy jumped up immediately and ran to his mother's arms shouting, 'Mummy, Mummy, there's a pony in here but I can't find him.'

Set Your Body Free

When it comes to physical strength and athletic prowess, juicing has real clout. After the Juice Blitz and ten days on the High Life Diet, your body becomes so much cleaner and clearer from inside out you no longer easily build up the wastes in the muscles and around joints that make exercisers and athletes so prone to injury. The kind of acidic buildup that comes with exercise is minimized, and you can work out longer and harder without pain. Replacing convenience foods with fresh foods and live juices also gradually stabilizes blood sugar so that energy for physical activity is readily available and long-lasting. After three months of juicing a marathon fell runner described it this way: 'Everything has become effortless. I can run longer and harder without straining. Instead of demanding so much of my will, I find myself almost floating over the hills and rocks. Just occasionally it gets so good, I feel as though I could run on forever.'

Fuel for Change

We believe that the benefits of Juice High have the potential to be felt far beyond the individual. Social change is brought about by the dreams, the visions, the thoughts and the actions of people. The greater the clarity of perception and an individual's sense of freedom, the more creativity and potential benefit he or she can bring to work, relationships and society as a whole. Our educational system – despite the high-sounding phrases bandied around by ministers – is dedicated not to turning out free-thinking, autonomous human beings but rather to 'normalizing' thought and behaviour. That way the status quo is maintained, and potent, active eccentrics whose visions go against the grain are kept in close check.

The goal of Juice High is diametrically opposed to this way of thinking. It is a potent tool for helping to establish freedom for each of us; the freedom to act according to our own perceptions and values and to pursue our own goals. These are goals which arise from the core of one's being rather than those which have been imposed from outside by parenting, schooling or the exploitative demands of our materialistic society.

Freedom is not, as advertisers would have us believe, drinking white rum on a tropical beach or wearing a pair of Levi 501s. Freedom is about living out the truth of your soul in the way you relate to others, in the work you do, in the creative pursuits and the choices you make. Of course such freedom is profoundly dangerous to those structures which would control us by delivering a pastiche of the real thing. Yet such freedom is the greatest high any of us ever experience – far better than any drug could offer. It is the freedom of learning to trust yourself.

Future Change

What is fascinating about real freedom is that it not only helps the individual experience and live out his or her own creativity, it also brings to our families, communities and the planet as a whole the very best that each of us has to offer.

Now, drinking a glass of green juice each morning and munching more carrots at lunch are not going to turn us into a Martin Luther King or a Mother Teresa. But they can go a long way towards helping us to clear away some of the physical, emotional and intellectual junk we have all picked up along the way that prevent us from being who we are, from seeing clearly, from trusting what we see and then acting on it. That is why we see *Juice High* as a practical, easy-to-use tool for personal transformation which can ultimately have a profoundly beneficial effect on the world around us. It is an exciting prospect.

Recipes

JUICE INDEX

There are several variables to be considered when formulating juice recipes. Fruit and vegetables have not yet been standardized (thank God) and vary considerably in size and juice yield. Not all centrifugal extractors are as efficient as others. Rather than give measurements in millilitres, we decided that the most practical way to present these recipes is by indicating roughly how many pieces of fruit and veg you'll need to make approximately 280ml/10 fl. oz/half a pint. Alas, Total Juices are made with a powerful blender rather than a centrifugal extractor.

Alfalfa – Father of all Juices
The word alfalfa means 'father of all grains' and when it comes to hair health you can't do better than alfalfa sprouts and carrot juice.

4–5 carrots
1 cup alfalfa sprouts
Chopped parsley (optional)

Juice as usual and top with some chopped parsley and drink.

Apples & Pears
Apples and pears are closely related and make a sublime combination when juiced together.

Juice High

2 *pears*
2 *whole apples*

Juice as usual and drink straight away as this oxidizes very quickly.

Apples, Celery & Fennel

2–3 *apples*
2 *stalks celery*
1 *bulb of fennel*

Apples, Pears & Berries

Berries are intensely-flavoured vitamin bombs that tend to be high in potassium and contain a remarkable range of other trace elements. Strawberries, raspberries, black-berries . . . in fact any berry works well when blended with apple juice, or apple and pear.

2 *apples*
1 *dozen berries (or as many as 1 pear you like)*

Reserve a couple of pieces of apple to put through the juicer last and to flush the thick berry juice through the machine.

Apple Zinger

A terrific breakfast-time enlivener that perks up the whole system and really wakes up your taste buds.

2 *or 3 whole apples*
1 *whole lemon, peeled*
1 *(or more) 1cm cube of ginger*

Atomic Lift-Off

This gives an immediate lift when you are feeling low. It's also a wonderful chaser for shots of tequila!

4–6 *ripe tomatoes*
1 *lime*
A *pinch of cayenne pepper, or dash of Tabasco*

Juice the tomatoes and the lime (removing the skin but leaving the pith) then sprinkle with a dash of cayenne pepper.

Beetroot, Carrot & Orange

Beetroot enriches the blood and provides an excellent tonic for the kidneys. The sweetness of orange juice in this recipe will help you become accustomed to the earthy flavour of beet.

1 smallish beet
4 carrots
1 orange

Save one of the carrots to put through the juicer last, as it will help to clear the machine.

Beet Treat

Profoundly powerful, this juice will give you sustained energy throughout the day.

½ whole beetroot (plus tops, if possible)
2 carrots
1 apple
1 stalk celery
3cm cucumber

Black Watermelon

You have two choices on how to prepare this, you can juice the skin of the watermelon as well as the pink flesh and then add the molasses and stir in. Or, you can take only the pink flesh, put it into a blender or food processor, add the molasses and blend. We prefer the second method but either is good.

¼ small watermelon
1 tsp–1 tbsp blackstrap molasses (unsulphured)

Carrot & Apple

This is the most basic juice cocktail; use it as the springboard for experimentation. Start by combining equal parts of the two juices and experiment until you find the proportions that suit you; we prefer one part apple to two parts carrot.

4 carrots
1 apple

Carrot & Orange

Peel the rind from oranges, but leave the pith, and put the whole fruit through the juicer together with the carrots.

1 orange
4 carrots

Carrot Milk

Adding soya milk to freshly-extracted carrot juice enhances its natural creaminess and gives you plenty of protein, without the clogging effect of cows' milk. Try adding the juice of a single small parsnip – scrubbed, topped and tailed but not peeled – and a little grated nutmeg.

3 carrots
1 parsnip
Soya milk to taste (or to fill the glass)

Carrot Milk (Total Juice)

2 carrots
1½ cups soya milk (see Resources, p. 432)
Pinch of nutmeg
Handful of ice cubes
Juice of ½ lemon
Pinch of nutmeg

Put carrots and soya milk into the blender with the ice cubes. Squeeze the lemon juice into the blender, blend for 30 seconds, top with fresh grated nutmeg and serve.

Carrot, Beet, Celery, Tomato

3 carrots
½ beetroot, peeled
2 stalks of celery
2 tomatoes

Carrot High

5 carrots
4 sticks celery
1 clove garlic

Celery Sticks

3–4 sticks celery
4–5 carrots
1 clove garlic

Juice as usual and drink immediately.

Chlorophyll Plus

A handful of dandelion leaves
A handful of parsley
A handful of spinach
1 whole apple
A small bunch of grapes

Citrus Carrot Special

This is a beautiful drink made even better if you chill all of the ingredients before you use them.

2 carrots (juiced)
½ small pineapple
1 small orange

Peel the orange and pineapple and cut into bite-sized pieces. Toss into the blender with a handful of ice cubes and the carrot juice. Blend and serve immediately.

Citrusucculent

1 ripe grapefruit (or pink grapefruit)
2 ripe oranges
½ ripe lemon
2 ripe oranges

Peel the fruit (leave the pith) and juice as usual.

Citrus Zinger

1 pink grapefruit
1 orange
½ lemon
½ lime
1 (or more) 1cm cube of ginger (optional)

Cool as a Cuke

1 cucumber
1 clove garlic
1 tomato
A dash of dill

Juice the vegetables and then sprinkle with ground dill and serve over ice.

Cranberry Cocktail

1 cup of cranberries
Lemon juice
1 cup of sweet grapes or 2–3 apples

Put the grapes or cranberries and apples through the juicer then add a squeeze of fresh lemon juice before serving. If you don't have fresh cranberries you can use frozen ones.

Dandelion Plus

4–5 carrots
A handful of dandelion leaves
1 bulb of fennel
Lemon juice

Juice as usual then add a tablespoon of lemon juice to the mixture.

Double Whammy

4–5 carrots
A handful of dandelion leaves
2 whole pears

Easy Does It

1 large green apple, whole
2 stalks celery
8–10 lettuce leaves

Juice as usual and drink before bedtime, or when you are feeling particularly tense.

Fab 5 Fruit Juice

A great fruit punch, this recipe can be varied and different fruits substituted according to seasonal availability.

½ apple
½ pear
1 tangerine, or similar
12 grapes
1 peach

Fatty Acid Frolic (Total Juice)

2 whole apples
2–3 dandelion leaves or large kale leaves or beetroot top
1 heaped tbsp of fresh vacuum-packed linseeds
1 very ripe banana

Juice the apple and leaves as usual. Put into a blender with the linseeds and the banana and blend at high speed until smooth. Drink immediately.

Fruit Frappé (Total Juice)

This is a lovely drink rather like a frozen Daiquiri. Whether or not you add alcohol to it is up to you.

½ banana
½ orange, pith left on
1 mango, peeled, with the inner peel removed
½ cup of frozen strawberries
½ cup of soya milk or low-fat yoghurt
A handful of ice cubes

Cut the fruit into easy-to-manage pieces (obviously peel the banana and the orange), toss into the blender with the ice cubes and blend for 30 seconds at high speed. Serve immediately.

Fruit Medley (Total Juice)

¼ small pineapple, peeled and cut into spears
1 small orange, peeled but with the pith left on
½ apple
½ banana
1 tbsp maple syrup or honey

Cut all the fruit into bite-sized pieces, place in the blender with a few ice cubes, turn on at high speed for half a minute. Serve immediately.

Ginger Berry

1 (or more) 1cm cube of fresh ginger
1 medium bunch of grapes
2 cups blackberries or raspberries

Juice as usual. You can also add some sparkling mineral water to this, or some ice; it makes a delicious and refreshing long drink on a hot day.

Gingeroo

Carrot and apple juice tastes even better if you ginger it up a little.

1 (or more) 1cm cube of fresh ginger
1 whole apple
4 carrots

Ginger's Best

½ cantaloupe melon
½ cm slice fresh ginger
1 lime (peel, leaving pith)

Ginger Spice

3 large carrots
1 whole pear
A small chunk of fresh ginger

Glorious Grapefruit

Apparently there is a world glut of pink grapefruits, which make a frothy, sweet and sharp juice that we love to drink for breakfast. Peel the fruit, but remember to leave as much of the white pith as possible to put through your juicer. Two grapefruits will yield slightly more than half a pint of juice.

Green Friend

3 whole apples
2–3 dandelion leaves or a couple of large kale leaves or
    beetroot top
A handful of mint

Green Goddess

This juice makes you smile like the Mona Lisa.

60ml (2 fl. oz) of carrot juice
60ml (2 fl. oz) of apple juice
60ml (2 fl. oz) of beetroot juice
60ml (2 fl. oz) of broccoli juice
½ tsp of kelp powder
½–1 tsp chopped fresh parsley
A squeeze of fresh lemon juice

Green Tomato

This invigorating green drink is not made with green tomatoes, which tend to be sour, but luscious red ones.

2–3 ripe tomatoes
2 stalks celery
1 green pepper
½ bulb of fennel
2–3 sprigs parsley/chopped parsley

Green Wild

2 whole green apples
2 stalks celery
½ lemon
1 (or more) 1cm cube of fresh ginger

Green Wow

2 green apples
4 stalks of celery
6 Chinese leaves
Juice of 10cm of cucumber

Green Zinger

2 kale leaves or beetroot tops or a handful of spinach
4–5 carrots
A small handful of parsley

Hi Mag

4–5 carrots
2 florets of broccoli
2 dandelion leaves, beetroot tops, spinach or kale leaves

Juice and season with a twist of lemon and a pinch of salt.

Hi NRG

1 apple
2 carrots
1 stalk of celery
Soya milk to taste

Hit the Grass (Total Juice)

A handful of fresh mint
A small pineapple, peeled and cut into convenient sized
  spears
A handful of any fresh cereal grass such as wheat or
  barley

Juice the mint and pineapple in your ordinary juicer, then juice the cereal grass in a wheat-grass juicer. Whisk together. Alternatively, pour the fruit juice into a food processor or blender and toss the cereal grasses in, blend with the blade until highly blended, then pour through a strainer to remove the indigestible fibre. Serve over ice. This can also be made using a teaspoon to a tablespoon of any of the freeze-dried cereal grasses such as barley grass or wheat grass.

Lazy Lettuce

2 whole apples
5 lettuce leaves

Lemon Zinger

1 whole apple
½ a lemon
Sparkling mineral water

Juice the apple and the lemon – leaving the white pith on the lemon – pour into a glass and top up with sparkling water and ice.

Leslie's Cocktail

Bananas are not totally unjuiceable if you use very ripe fruit. Put them through your juicer first, then the apples, which will help to flush the thick banana through the machine. Alternatively, use a blender to make the breakfast of champions. This recipe also works well with melon in place of apple.

180ml (6 fl. oz) of fresh apple juice
1 ripe banana
1 tsp each of spirulina, chlorella, and green barley powder

Linusit Perfect

This recipe is replete with valuable essential fatty acids – both omega-6 and omega-3 – which are often deficient in people who have been surviving on the typical Western fare of convenience foods. It must be made with freshly ground vacuum-packed linseeds or flaxseeds for these precious fatty acids are highly unstable and go rancid quickly.

2 whole apples
½cm slice of ginger
3 carrots
1 tbsp linseeds or flaxseeds

Juice the fruit, carrots and ginger as usual. Place the linseed in a coffee grinder and grind finely. Then add to the glass of juice, stir well and drink immediately. Alternatively you can put the linseed into a food processor, grind and then pour the freshly made juice in and blend for 3 seconds.

Merry Belon

Berries are one kind of fruit that combines really well with melons and the array of flavours gives lots of scope for experimentation. Try galia & raspberry, honeydew & blackberry or the classic watermelon & strawberry.

1 slice of watermelon, 3 cm wide and cut into chunks to
  fit your juicer
6 strawberries, washed and with their green stalks
  removed

In hot weather, a good tip is to freeze the berries before juicing them.

More Raw NRG

Like the Raw NRG cocktail, More Raw is based on the crucial combination of carrot and apple, with green vegetable juices diluted by cucumber and celery. When making this juice, put the ingredients through your juicer in reverse order and you'll end up with a greenish drink tinged with orange froth.

3 carrots
1 apple
2 stalks of celery
3 cm section of cucumber
1 broccoli floret
A small bunch of spinach or watercress (or dandelion
  leaves)

Orange Tonic

2 oranges
1 (or more) 1cm cube of fresh ginger
Sparkling water

Juice the ginger and orange as usual, pour into a glass and top up with sparkling mineral water. This is particularly delicious in winter.

Papaya & Pineapple

This exotic combination is especially good for settling upset stomachs.

½ small pineapple, cut into spears
1 mango

Take care to remove all the flesh from the stone of the mango before you juice it.

Parsley Passion

Another vegetable rich in mineral salts is parsley. Drinking parsley juice daily can bring relief to people troubled by allergies.

1 bunch parsley
3–5 carrots
2 apples
2 small cauliflower florets

Parsnip Perfect

Parsnips, also know as anaemic carrots, are well known for their ability to strengthen hair, skin and nails and can protect against hair loss.

2 parsnips
3 carrots
1 beetroot

Pepper Upper

This juice is a great replacement for tea breaks and mid-afternoon pick-me-ups of coffee and biscuits. It helps you to sizzle with vitality without any of the downside you get from sugar and caffeine.

2 carrots
1 red pepper
1 stick celery
¼ bunch of watercress
2–3 sprigs of parsley

Save one of the carrots until last to clear out any juice left inside your machine. Otherwise, put the ingredients through in any order, stir and serve.

Pineamint

Especially good if taken at bedtime for settling the stomach and helping you sleep.

1 small pineapple
A small bunch of fresh mint leaves

Remove the skin of the pineapple and cut into convenient spears. Juice as usual and serve over ice for a long summer drink.

Pineappage

This may seem like a weird combination, but it's one way to sweeten the mega-nutrient fix of fresh cabbage.

¼ large pineapple cut into spears
⅓ green cabbage

Pineapple Grapefruit Drink

1 small pineapple
1 peeled grapefruit

Pineapple Green

To 180ml (6 fl. oz) of freshly extracted pineapple juice add one or more of the following:

*1 tsp–1 tbsp of powdered wheat grass, green barley,
   spirulina or chlorella*

Popeye Punch

1 whole apple – including seeds
4 or 5 carrots
A small handful of spinach
1 cucumber

Potassium Power (Total Juice)

*1 yellow or green melon, such as cantaloupe, honeydew
   etc.*
1 over-ripe banana
A pinch of grated nutmeg
6 cubes ice (made with spring water)

Scoop out the flesh of the melon, place in a food processor or blender, add the banana, blend well, pour into a glass over the ice cubes and sprinkle with a pinch of freshly ground nutmeg.

Potassium Punch

Our tribute to N.W.Walker, the American raw food pioneer and evangelist of detoxification; drink it religiously!

3 carrots
2 stalks celery
4–6 leaves of lettuce or winter greens
A few stalks of fresh coriander or parsley
*A handful of spinach or watercress (or dandelion
   leaves)*

Pulp Gazpacho (Total Juice)

You can also make wonderful raw soups as well as uncooked warm soups using total juicing methods.

2 cups of spring water
1 medium sized carrot
1 stick celery
2 spring onions
4 ripe tomatoes, chilled
1 tsp Marigold Swiss vegetable bouillon powder (see Resources, p. 432)
A dash of white wine
1 tsp parsley

Place all the ingredients in the blender. Add two or three ice cubes, blend for 30 seconds, sprinkle with parsley and serve.

Quantum Green (Total Juice)

A super-charged blender drink enriched with sprouted pulses and sunflower seeds. Apples can be substituted for the pineapple.

3 carrots
2 spears of pineapple
¼ cup soaked sunflower seeds
¼ cup assorted sprouts
A handful of spinach leaves

Juice the spinach with the carrots, then cut the pineapple into chunks and put into the blender with the sprouts and seeds. Blend together, adding the freshly made juice.

Raw NRG

Carrot and apple juice is the basis for this health-packed cocktail, which is devised to promote all-round health with the addition of celery and cucumber to the carrot and apple base. As you become more adventurous in your juicing, try reducing the apple content and adding green leaves of cabbage, spinach or dandelion to increase the green energy content.

1 apple
4 carrots
1 or 2 stalks of celery
5cm section of cucumber
1cm cube of fresh ginger (optional)

The addition of a cube or two of ginger gives the Raw NRG mix a real zing.

Red Cool

The addition of a cube or more of ginger makes Red Cool red hot.

1 beetroot
2 apples
4 carrots
1 (or more) 1cm cube of fresh ginger

Red Devil

This recipe provides a real tonic for the blood and is a great source of vitamins A, B-complex, C, D, beta-carotene, vitamins K and E as well as calcium, iron, potassium, magnesium, manganese, sulphur, iodine and copper. It's also useful for clearing infections of the urinary tract and upset stomachs.

3 carrots
3 stalks celery
1 beetroot

Put the carrots and celery in the juicer first and then add the beetroot. If feeling extravagant, serve with half a teaspoon of fresh cream floated on the top.

Red Flag

3 small ripe tomatoes
4 carrots
A handful of spinach

Red Genius

4 carrots
1 large raw beetroot
3cm section of cucumber

Rhubarb Radiance

Drink at night before bed.

2 large stalks rhubarb
3 medium apples

Roots Soup

Root vegetables are the best source of B-complex vitamins. Here, their thick, sweet and creamy juices are complemented by the aniseed flavour of fennel. Dilute your roots soup with cucumber juice, but if it's still too thick add a splash of spring water.

½ smallish beetroot
1 medium-sized parsnip
1 sweet potato
½ bulb of fennel
5cm section of cucumber

Salad Juice

4–5 carrots
4 sticks celery
3–4 radishes

Salsa Surprise

2 large ripe tomatoes
3 carrots
2 sticks celery
A small bunch of parsley
1 clove garlic

Scary Mary

See Virgin Mary

Secret of the Sea (Total Juice)

4 carrots
2 whole apples
2 sheets nori seaweed

Juice the apple and carrot then pour into a blender along with the seaweed. Blend thoroughly and serve. This is even better if you toast the seaweed under a grill or near a flame or hotplate, very briefly – it takes no more than 10 or 15 seconds to do on both sides. You can then break it up into the juice and blend.

Silky Strawberries (Total Juice)

Strawberries are surprisingly potent when it comes to supporting a body that is under stress. Just 100gms of strawberries contain as much as 80mg vitamin C, as well as all the other vitamins except for B12 and D, plus valuable minerals. Strawberries have a natural diuretic action and are very calming to the liver. They also contain salicylic acid which, according to experts in natural medicine, is good for any sort of kidney or joint complaint.

2 cups strawberries
1 ripe pear
1 ripe banana
A handful of fresh mint leaves

Juice the strawberries and pear as usual then place in a blender with the banana and mint and blend until smooth. This drink is particularly delicious when made with a frozen banana; it takes on the taste and consistency of a natural ice-cream.

Smooth as Silk (Total Juice)

This recipe is rich in natural fruit sugars, potassium, magnesium and the amino acid tryptophan which can be turned into serotonin in the brain. It is also absolutely irresistible.

2 cups blackberries, either fresh or frozen
1 whole banana
1 ripe apple

Juice the berries and the apple. Put the juice and banana into a food processor or blender and blend until smooth. Drink 45 minutes before bedtime.

Spicy Apple

2 apples, whole
1 lime
A pinch of cinnamon

Juice the apples and the lime (leave the pith on the lime), sprinkle with cinnamon and serve.

Spicy Carrot

This juice is a great source of minerals such as magnesium, potassium, calcium, iron, sulphur, copper, phosphorus and iodine, as well as anti-oxidants, beta-carotene, vitamins A, C, E and niacin, vitamins D and K. It will also soothe a delicate stomach. Braeburn and Cox's are ideal for this juice, but any sweet apple will do.

Juice High

4 carrots
2 spears of pineapple
1 Braeburn or Cox's apple
A pinch of ground cinnamon
A pinch of ground nutmeg

Pineapples vary considerably in size. You'll need half a small one or a quarter of a big one. Remove the fibrous skin with a sharp knife and cut into long spears that will fit into your juicer. The cinnamon and nutmeg can be sprinkled on top of the freshly-extracted juice, or stirred into it as you prefer.

Spiked Celery

4 stalks celery
4–5 carrots
1 clove garlic

Spinapple

When you mix apple with spinach you have an amazing combination for cleansing the digestive tract and improving elimination quickly, probably because spinach (which is high in oxalic acid) combines with the pectin in the apple's mineral salts to form a unique compound that has remarkable cleansing actions. Some practitioners in natural medicine claim that it actually clears old encrusted faeces that has accumulated over months and years in the colon making it possible to eliminate it from the body.

3 whole apples
A handful of spinach

Drink twice a day; especially important just before bedtime.

Spring Salad

3 florets of broccoli
4 carrots
2 stalks of celery
1 clove of garlic
1 tomato

Sprouting o' the Green

2 cups of alfalfa sprouts
2 cups of mung-bean sprouts
1 carrot
A few sprigs of parsley
2 apples

Sprout Special

This juice is rich in natural phyto-hormones that help protect the body from the damage that petrochemically derived pesticides and herbicides can foster. It is also enormously rich in life-enhancing enzymes.

4 carrots
1 whole apple
1 cup sprouted seeds (mung beans, alfalfa, chickpeas, adzuki beans, etc)

Sprinkle some grated ginger on top or a little cinnamon and serve over ice.

Straight CJ

When buying carrots, choose those with the darkest colour. Size doesn't matter, but many of the recipes in this book refer to 'medium-sized' carrots, around 15cm in length. Whichever variety you use, you'll need about a pound, or half a kilo of carrots to make 280ml or 10fl.oz juice. As a rule of thumb, we reckon that half a dozen medium carrots will yield about half a pint of juice. Scrub them under cold running water and remove the tops and tails, but it is not necessary to peel carrots before putting them through the juicer.

Sweet and Spicy

2 whole apples
2 x 1cm cube fresh ginger
½ small pineapple cut into convenient-sized spears

Juice as usual, adding as much ginger as you like, and sprinkle with a little ground cinnamon.

Sweet Salvation

Sweet capsicums (peppers) contain more vitamin C than oranges. Here, the juice is blended with freshly-made tomato juice to produce a deep red-orange, sweet yet savoury drink.

1 red or yellow pepper
2 ripe tomatoes (or 1 beef tomato)
3cm section of cucumber
1–2 carrots

Tomato & Carrot, Celery & Lime

A deliciously light combination (and not a bad medium for pepper vodka):

2–3 ripe tomatoes
2 carrots
2 stalks of celery
½ lime

Top of the Beet

1 apple
5 carrots
3 leaves of beetroot top
A handful of parsley

Tossled Carrot

5 big carrots
1 whole apple
A pinch of turmeric

Juice the carrots and apple, pour into glasses and sprinkle with turmeric.

Tropical Prune

1 small pineapple, peeled and cut into convenient-sized
  spears
2 fresh prunes – when prunes are not in season, substitute
  one pear

Juice as normal, then grate a pinch of nutmeg on to the top and serve.

Vegetarian

4 carrots
½ bulb of fennel
1 apple
1 lime
Either a handful of fresh cereal grass or 1 tsp–1 tbsp
  powdered green supplements

Juice all ingredients except for the cereal grasses, then put the juice and the cereal grasses in a blender or food processor and blend thoroughly. Strain before serving to remove the indigestible fibre. If you use a powdered green supplement as well, then juice as normal, pour the juice into the food processor or blender, add the powdered green supplement, blend and serve over ice.

Vampire Mary

See Virgin Mary, below.

Virgin Mary

A Bloody Mary without the vodka, we find that the flavour of this refreshing tomato-based cocktail benefits from a few drops of Tabasco. Add a clove of garlic and it becomes a Vampire Mary; a fresh jalapeno or other hot green chilli pepper turns it into a Scary Mary.

2 ripe tomatoes
2 carrots
½ beetroot
1 stalk celery
1 cucumber

Waterfall

5cm section of cucumber
1 whole apple
3 carrots
½ smallish beetroot

HIGH LIFE RECIPES: SALADS

Trio Salads

Trio Salads are best of all. The principles of making them are simple. Mix together three vegetables – one root, one bulb (or 'fruit') vegetable, and one leaf vegetable. Garnish with fresh or dried herbs and add dressing.

Root vegetables: carrots, celeriac, turnips, onions, leeks, beetroot, radishes, white radishes, etc.

Bulb or 'fruit' vegetables: tomatoes, red and green peppers, fennel, avocado, cucumber, cauliflower, celery, broccoli, courgettes, mushrooms, calabrese, etc.

Leaf vegetables: lettuce, young dandelion leaves, young beet tops, red or white cabbage, Brussels sprouts, spring onions, spring greens, spinach, chicory, endive, etc. Watercress, cress and sprouted grains and seeds can be used in any combination, or on their own, or as a garnish.

To increase a salad's protein content you can sprinkle it with three-seed mixture, an excellent source of both omega-3 and omega-6 essential fatty acids. Mix together equal quantities of sunflower, pumpkin and sesame seeds, grind in a coffee grinder, then sprinkle on the salad. Three-seed mixture can also be added to breakfasts and to drinks. Once ground it should be stored in the refrigerator. You can also give salads a protein lift with mixed nuts, or sprouted seeds or grains, or add some soft goat's cheese, free-range chicken, chopped boiled eggs, prawns, etc.

Sprout Salad

Mix two or three kinds of sprouted grains or seeds (a handful of each) in a bowl, add half a sliced avocado and season with fresh basil and chives. Garnish with black olives and dress with garlic dressing.

Spinach Splendour

2 cups spinach
1 cup fresh mushrooms

Remove stems and veins of spinach. Slice mushrooms finely and mix together. Toss in garlic dressing and sprinkle with basil or sunflower seeds.

Red Slaw

1½ cups grated cabbage
1 grated carrot
½ grated green pepper
1 tbsp honey
A pinch of celery seeds

Toss with salad dressing and serve.

Sunshine Salad

The fresh pineapple gives this salad a tropical taste. Make sure your pineapple is ripe by pulling out one of its centre leaves; if it comes out easily it is ready to eat.

A few crisp lettuce leaves
1 fresh pineapple
2 carrots
2 sticks celery
½ green pepper
2 handfuls of sultanas (or raisins)
½ tsp celery seeds
1 tsp dry mustard mixed with vinaigrette

Wash and crisp the lettuce leaves in the fridge. Peel the pineapple (it is not necessary to core it) and cut it into fairly small cubes. Coarsely grate the carrots, and finely chop the celery and green pepper, and add them to the pineapple cubes. Add the sultanas, soaked in water for a few hours to plump them up. Sprinkle with celery seeds and serve on a bed of crisp lettuce leaves. Serve with a piquant mustardy mayonnaise or French dressing.

Orange Orange Salad

A surprising combination . . . but it works!

4 carrots
6 oranges
1–2 cups white cabbage
2 handfuls of raisins or small seedless grapes
4 tsp sesame seeds

Coarsely chop the carrots. Juice four of the oranges and blend the juice with the carrots until you have a smooth mixture. Finely shred or grate the cabbage and put it in a bowl with the raisins or grapes. Pour the carrot mixture over it and lightly mix with a fork. Sprinkle with the sesame seeds and garnish with the two remaining oranges, peeled and sliced.

Summer Symphony

This salad is an exciting play of colours and shapes – the more variety the better.

1 lettuce (cos is good)
1 cup small cauliflower florets
2 celery stalks (finely chopped)
2 carrots (finely grated or cut into matchsticks)
6 cherry tomatoes
4 radishes (sliced)
1 green pepper (cut into thin strips)
Watercress
Fresh sweetcorn or alfalfa sprouts to garnish

Place the lettuce leaves, torn into bite-sized pieces or shredded, into a bowl – a clear glass bowl is nice for this one so that all the beautiful colours show through it. Prepare the vegetables and arrange in layers in the bowl, keeping the watercress for decoration. Dress with a thinned mayonnaise dressing, perhaps blended with a tomato or two, and top with sweet corn or alfalfa sprouts, and sprigs of watercress.

Sprout Magic Salad

Make a base with alfalfa or mung sprouts and around the dish arrange:

grated carrot
red cabbage
white cabbage
beetroot
sliced mushrooms
black olives
spring onions

Sprinkle raisins over the grated vegetables and spoon over a rich dressing.

SALAD DRESSINGS

Basic Dressing

Mix one part lemon juice and two parts extra virgin olive oil or four parts mashed avocado. Add herbs, garlic, mustard or honey to this base.

Tomato Dressing

3–5 tomatoes
2 tbsp lemon juice
½ tsp basil

Put into a blender and liquefy. Store in the fridge.

Avocado-Tomato Dressing

4 small tomatoes
1 avocado
2 tbsp lemon juice
A dash of Tabasco
1 crushed clove of garlic or a dash of garlic powder

Mix in a blender. Store in the fridge.

Yoghurt and Egg Dressing

1 egg yolk
1½ cups non-fat yoghurt
3 tbsp lemon juice or cider vinegar
A pinch of cayenne pepper
Fresh or dried herbs to taste
2 tsp honey

Put the ingredients into the top of a double boiler and stir over hot water until the mixture thickens. Refrigerate to serve cold or use hot, on hot potato salad or hot rice salad.

Thousand Island Dressing

1 hard-boiled egg, chopped
5 tsp celery, finely chopped
3 tbsp onion, finely chopped
2 tbsp black olives, chopped
1 tbsp green pepper, finely chopped
½ cup non-fat yoghurt

Mix all the ingredients together and serve chilled.

Non-Oil Vinaigrette

3 tbsp dried skimmed milk
½ tsp Dijon mustard
2 tsp honey
A dash of pepper
A pinch of basil
1 clove garlic, crushed
2 tbsp vinegar

Mix the ingredients, adding the vinegar last. Beat well or blend until smooth. Chill and use the same day.

RAW SOUPS

Cucumber

1 cup low-fat yoghurt or soya milk
½ cucumber, peeled and sliced
A sprig of mint
1 tsp lemon juice

Blend and serve sprinkled with parsley.

Gazpacho (see also Pulp Gazpacho, p. 305)

4–6 peeled tomatoes
3 carrots
2 sticks of celery
A dash of cayenne

Put through a juicer, sprinkle with chopped chives and diced green pepper.

Avocado Smoothie

¾ cup low-fat yoghurt or tofu
½ avocado
¼ diced red pepper
1 tsp lemon juice
1 chopped spring onion
A dash of Tabasco

Blend and serve.

Carrot Chowder

1 cup nuts (almonds, hazels or pecans)
1 cup low-fat yoghurt
2 egg yolks
1 tbsp olive oil
Small clove of garlic
Juice of ½ lemon

2 tsp vegetable bouillon powder (see Resources, page 432)
3 cups carrot juice (using about 12 big carrots)
Ice cubes
½ green pepper
2 spring onions
Chopped parsley

Grind the nuts finely and blend them with the yoghurt, egg yolks, pressed garlic, lemon juice, olive oil and seasoning. Juice the carrots into a jar with ice cubes in it, then slowly add the juice and ice to the yoghurt mixture, stirring well. Serve sprinkled with a mixture of finely chopped green pepper, spring onion and parsley.

Flamingo Soup

2 medium-sized beetroot
10 carrots
1 small head celery
Ice
Juice of 1 lemon
4–6 tomatoes
2 handfuls almonds
1 tbsp fresh thyme
1 tbsp fresh basil
Marigold Swiss vegetable bouillon powder (see Resources, p. 432) to taste
6 tbsp yoghurt
Chives

Juice the beetroot, carrots and celery and put into an airtight jar with some ice and the lemon juice. Blend the tomatoes, almonds, thyme, basil and bouillon powder. Combine the two mixtures and serve in bowls with a spoonful of yoghurt and a sprinkling of chopped chives.

Fresh Green Soup

2 avocados, peeled and stoned
3 cups apple juice
Juice of ½ lemon
1 courgette
A handful of alfalfa and mung sprouts
1 stick celery
Parsley
2 tsp tamari
1 tsp Marigold Swiss vegetable bouillon powder (see
  Resources, p. 432)
Ground ginger
Sliced mushrooms or flaked almonds

Combine the avocados, apple juice, lemon juice, parsley, tamari, vegetable bouillon and a pinch of ginger in the blender. Grate the courgette and finely dice the celery and mix them with the sprouts. Now pour on the avocado sauce. Serve sprinkled with sliced mushroom or flakes of almond.

MUESLI

Live Muesli

1–2 tbsp breakfast oats, soaked overnight in a little
  spring water
1 grated apple (or mango, peach, strawberries, etc)
½ cup low-fat yoghurt

Mix all the ingredients and sprinkle with toasted seeds or mixed nuts.

PARTY TIME

Raw juices are seriously good for you. But who wants to be serious all the time? Not only is it OK to have fun, but making time to relax and enjoy yourself is crucial. Raw juices are not just for the abstemious and self-consciously healthy; they're also utterly delicious and appeal to the hedonist inside all of us.

Naturally sweet, fruity drinks are the healthy alternative to sugary pop that usually fuels children's parties and tends to make kids hyperactive, not to say stroppy. We can't guarantee that your child's birthday party won't end in tears if you give the young guests raw juice instead of fizzy drinks and fruit smoothies instead of ice cream sundaes, but our experience suggests that children will get a lot less fractious and play more happily together if you do.

Not that there is anything childish about the kind of fruit punches suggested in this section. Mixed with alcohol, freshly extracted juices make the most seductive cocktails and are guaranteed to make any social gathering flow easily. Which is not to suggest that getting intoxicated on a regular basis is a great idea, but that the expansive conviviality induced by alcohol helps us all to remember that we're only human.

Raw juices make the most sublime mixers for alcohol, but at any adult gathering there will be a proportion of people who do not wish to drink alcohol. Raw juice is a great leveller at parties because you can devise cocktails that taste just as good with or without a shot of alcohol. Teetotallers and hardcore hedonists can then mingle with impunity, all cradling glasses that look the same.

The first time we observed this phenomenon was at a marathon poetry performance for which we concocted a Purple Poetry Potion. It being an evening of beat poetry reading we used beetroot juice, mixed with apple and pear, with or without vodka. Beat poets have varying needs. Some wanted a stiff drink to steady their nerves; others were in rehab and scrupulously avoided stiff drinks. All, however, were intrigued by the profoundly earthy potion and some were moved to new heights of lyricism!

SMOOTHIES

Children of all ages love smoothies, made in a blender rather than a juicer, which is particularly appropriate for liquefying bananas. Bananas *are* juiceable if you use very soft specimens and follow them through your juicer with very watery fruits such as melons, which will help to wash the thick banana through the machine. However, using a blender to make banana drinks is a lot easier and less wasteful.

Many soft exotic fruits including peaches and mangoes, papaya and pineapple work well in the blender (so long as you take care to remove all their skin and stones). Smoothies are especially good when blended with plain yoghurt, which give them the texture of milk shakes, or melted ice cream with a low fat content. Use low-fat yoghurt, or Greek yoghurt made with goats' milk. These are a few of our favourite combinations:

Banana & Pineapple Smoothie

1 banana
2 spears of pineapple
3 tbsp low-fat yoghurt

Peel the banana and break into chunks. Remove the fibrous skin from the pineapple and cut into spears, then into chunks. Put all the ingredients into the blender and blend until smooth.

Mango & Peach Smoothie

If you have a problem getting the stone out of a mango, the trick is to use a tablespoon. Cut around the edge of the fruit with a sharp knife. Slide the spoon over one side of the stone and twist it.

1 mango
3 peaches
3 tbsp low-fat yoghurt

Stone the mango and the peaches and cut both fruits into chunks. Put all the ingredients into the blender and blend until smooth.

Banana & Peach Smoothie with Strawberries

1 banana
1 peach
12 strawberries
3 tbsp low-fat yoghurt

Peel the banana and break it up into chunks. Remove the stone from the peach and chop it into chunks. Remove the green stalks from the strawberries. Put all the ingredients into the blender and blend until smooth.

Cantaloupe & Papaya Smoothie

Cantaloupe melons, with their rough skins and flesh of a delicate pink, orange or green colour, produce a rich, sweet juice that blends well with other exotic fruits.

½ cantaloupe melon
1 papaya

Cut the melon into spears, remove the flesh from the skin. Peel the papaya and scrape out the seeds. Chop both into chunks, put into the blender and blend until smooth. You can use mango instead of papaya and you may also like to add a piece of citrus fruit – an orange, or maybe a lime – to add another dimension.

Banana & Honeydew with Apricot

A mild, quite thick nectar that is best served over ice, or thinned with a splash of spring water. Less than half a honeydew should be more than adequate. Cut the melon into spears, then slice the flesh into chunks and remove from the skin.

1 banana
⅓ honeydew melon
6 apricots

Peel the banana, stone the apricots and remove the flesh from the melon. Put all the ingredients into a blender and blend until smooth.

EXOTIC FRUIT COCKTAILS

International commerce has blurred the seasons so that there is an abundant supply of exotic fruits in the supermarkets all year round, but summer is the right time to make the most of them. Exotic fruity cocktails made with a centrifugal juice extractor have an amazingly creamy texture and are perfect refreshment for a hot afternoon. For garden parties and barbecues, they're ideal.

The recipe suggestions below could be enlivened with the addition of a jigger of rum, or maybe a splash of vodka: far be it for us to discourage experimentation. The ideal way to chill these drinks is with a handful of crushed ice in the bottom of each glass, but it's also a good idea to keep all the ingredients refrigerated or iced in an insulated box.

Melon Medley with Berries

You can mix different kinds of melon juice together to create sublime blends, such as Honeyloupe (cantaloupe and honeydew, which is even better with a hint of ginger). Add summer berries to perk up their flavour. Use this recipe as the basis for experimentation.

1 slice watermelon
1 slice honeydew
12 raspberries

Peel the waxy outer skin from the honeydew and wash the rind of the watermelon. Juice the ingredients together and serve over ice.

Cantaloupe and Carrot with a Twist of Lemon

An intriguing and refreshing combination with a marvellous colour.

½ cantaloupe melon
3 carrots
½ lemon

Remove the rind from the melon with a vegetable peeler and the skin from the lemon, leaving the pith. Juice together, leaving one of the carrots to put through your juicer last.

Kiwi and Grape with Honeydew

Kiwis do not have to be peeled before juicing, so long as they're thoroughly washed. They have a slightly sharp flavour that blends well with melon and this juice is light, green and refreshing.

2 kiwi fruits
¼ honeydew melon
12 green grapes

Peel the waxy rind from the melon and put the flesh through the juicer with the other ingredients.

Orangeade

Forget about proprietary canned drinks and make your own sparkling summer cooler.

2 oranges
¼ lemon
¼ lime
Soda or sparkling spring water

Peel the citrus fruits, leaving on the white pith, and serve, topping up the glass with soda or sparkling water.

Orange & Raspberry

A terrific, summery combination with an amazing colour.

2 oranges (about 12)
A handful of raspberries

Peel the oranges, leaving on the pith, and juice as usual with the raspberries.

Pinorange

Pineapple and orange is a great, refreshing combination. Oranges vary considerably in juiciness: you'll need one big, firm, luscious orange or two smaller specimens.

2 spears of pineapple (about ½ a smallish fruit)
1 or 2 oranges

Peel the fibrous outer skin from the pineapple and the waxy skin from the orange, leaving the pith. Juice together.

THE ALCOHOL CONNECTION

The juices used in most cocktail bars come out of a carton and are rarely fresh, but you can set up a raw juice bar to make drinks that taste superb and are nourishing as well as intoxicating! Raw juice is especially useful for mixing with the clear spirits, particularly vodka, but be careful how much you add, since raw juice cocktails are deceptively easy to drink. Remember the golden rule of moderation in all things.

Cocktails were originally invented during Prohibition in America to disguise the harsh taste of illegally-distilled hooch. However, we never touch cheap liquor and recommend that you stick to the more refined premium brands, which have been distilled to a higher specification and will leave you with less of a hangover.

The exception to the quality rule is when mixing juices with sparkling wine to make the ultimate party punch. Using real Champagne is an unnecessary extravagance when there is now such a variety of good, cheap sparkling wines from Spain and the New World on the market. Here are a few of our favourite sparklers:

Mimosa/Bellini/Tiziano

Mimosa, or Buck's Fizz, is a simple half and half mixture of Champagne and orange juice. The same drink made with peaches, or apricots is a Bellini; one made with red grapes is a Tiziano. A tip is to add the juice to the sparkling wine, which will reduce the over-frothing that tends to happen if you try it the other way round.

Champagne Cooler

½ small pineapple
1 lemon
Sparkling wine

Half fill a tall glass with ice. Juice the fruit and pour it over the ice, then top with sparkling wine.

Mango/Papaya Go-Go

Use either mango or papaya to make this unusual and startlingly good party fuel.

1 large, ripe mango or papaya
2 kiwi fruits
1 big carrot
Sparkling wine

Remove the flesh from the mango, or peel and seed the papaya. Juice with the kiwi fruit and the carrot. Pour into a glass, stir and top with sparkling wine.

Sangria Real

Possibly the most popular summer party drink, Sangria, made with freshly extracted fruit juices mixed with red wine and given a sparkle with a splash of soda is an unbeatable way to relax on a hot day.

1 orange
¼ lemon
½ lime
Red wine
Soda or sparkling spring water

Half fill a tall glass with ice and pour in a wineglass measure of red wine. Leaving the pith on the citrus fruits, juice them and pour over the red wine and enough soda or sparkling mineral water to fill the glass. Stir and drink through a straw.

MARGARITA TIME

Distilled from the fermented juice of an Agave cactus, tequila is most often drunk in the form of a Margarita. The classic Margarita is made with lime juice and Cointreau and served in a salt-rimmed glass, but frozen margaritas, like alcoholic slush puppies, have become ubiquitous. If you have a masticating juicer, like the Champion (see Resources. p. 432), you can make excellent frozen Margaritas simply by freezing the fruit before you put it through the juicer. If using a centrifugal extractor, freezing the fruit will reduce its juice yield, but will chill the drink.

Strawberry Margarita

If you can find a blood orange to make your Margarita, so much the better.

60ml (2 fl.oz) tequila
12 frozen strawberries
1 orange
½ lime

Measure the tequila into a glass. Juice the fruit in the order listed and pour over the tequila. Serve.

RUM-BASED DRINKS

Rum, made from molasses, is ideally suited to mixing with fruit juices. Bacardi – a blend of white rums from different countries – is the single biggest alcohol brand in the world, but many tropical islands produce their own brands of rum and each has its own characteristics although some, such as Wray & Nephew's overproof white rum are pretty hard to take unless heavily diluted. Experiment, also, with darker rums like Myers, Cockspur and even Bacardi Gold.

Piña Colada

The classic tropical cocktail. You can buy coconut cream in cans or, as a last resort, use one of the proprietary brands like Malibu, which is ready-mixed with rum.

Juice High

2 *spears of pineapple*
3 *large tablespoons (75ml) coconut cream*
60ml *(2 fl.oz) white rum*
1 *Maraschino cherry*

Serve over crushed ice, garnished with a Maraschino cherry on top.

Rum Punch

Not a Planters' Punch, which is made with simple syrup and flavoured with lime and Angostura, but a long, exotic, slightly fizzy drink. Use the biggest, ripest mangoes you can lay your hands on.

1 *mango*
½ *lemon*
1 *lime*
60ml *(2 fl.oz) dark rum*
Soda water

Juice the mango and the citrus fruits, leaving on the white pith. Put some crushed ice into a glass and pour the rum over it. Pour in the fruit juices, stir, and top with a splash of soda.

Euphoria

Curaçao is a West Indian liquor made from bitter oranges (originally from the island of Curaçao) which is now available in a range of colours. The original remains best for this recipe.

½ *pink grapefruit*
1 *spear pineapple*
60ml *(2 fl.oz) white rum*
15ml *(½ fl.oz) Curaçao*

Measure the alcohol into a glass half-filled with crushed ice. Juice the grapefruit and pineapple and stir into the rum. The Curaçao can be floated on top of the drink or stirred into it.

VODKA-BASED DRINKS

Vodka is increasingly popular, particularly with people who don't like the taste of alcohol, because it has little or no flavour and can easily be disguised by mixing with fruit juices. We prefer to use a premium brand, such as Absolut, which is exceptionally pure and won't give you a hangover. When travelling, seek out the extra-strength, red label Absolut in duty-free shops.

Harvey Wallbanger

A screwdriver, vodka mixed with orange juice, is the most basic vodka cocktail. This is a more sophisticated variation, with the addition of a spoonful of Galliano, the spicy, herby Italian liquor that's sold in tall bottles, floated on top.

1 large, ripe orange
60ml (2 fl.oz) vodka
1 tbsp of Galliano

Measure the vodka into a glass, over ice. Juice the orange and mix it in. Gently float the Galliano on top.

Lucky Jim

A longer version of this classic variation of the Dry Martini, this recipe makes a light green, refreshing cocktail. A great aperitif, this recipe also works well with gin.

3cm section of cucumber
1 stalk of celery
60ml (2 fl.oz) vodka
A splash of dry vermouth (such as Noilly Prat)

Put some ice cubes in the bottom of a tall glass and add a splash of vodka. Leave to stand while juicing the cucumber and celery. Add the juice and the vodka, stir and serve with a stalk of parsley to garnish.

Ultimate Bloody Mary

There must be more recipes for Bloody Mary than for any other mixed drink, but most are predicated on canned tomato juice and require wakening-up with a dash of sherry and a range of garnishes. This one uses raw juice and doesn't require such extraneous adornments, unless you are partial to them.

3 ripe tomatoes
1 stalk celery
5 cm section of cucumber
60 ml (2 fl.oz) vodka
A dash of Tabasco, or Worcestershire Sauce
Salt and cayenne pepper or grated horseradish

Measure the vodka over ice. Juice the remaining ingredients, stir and serve with your choice of seasonings.

BOOK THREE:
RAW ENERGY RECIPES

For Joyce Pearce who makes
the best Raw Energy Cuisine
in the Southern Hemisphere

Contents

Introduction

For someone who's never experienced it before there can seem something magical about a high-raw diet. A way of eating in which about 50 to 75 per cent of your foods are taken uncooked increases your vitality, makes you look and feel great, and even helps protect from degenerative illness and premature ageing. Uncooked foods such as fresh crisp vegetables and luscious fruits, natural unprocessed seeds, grains and nuts have a quality of energy which is light yet strong and extraordinarily health-giving. They impart a similar power to the person eating them. Such foods are the richest natural sources of vitamins, minerals and enzymes you will find – all of which are important for high-level health – as well as good-quality protein, easily assimilated complex carbohydrates and essential fatty acids. They are also an excellent source of unadulterated natural fibre.

A high-raw diet has been used in some of Europe's finest clinics for over a hundred years – to cure illness, to increase vitality, to rejuvenate the body, to improve athletic performance, to beautify, and to encourage natural weight loss. It is such a diet that keeps world-famous health spas making money hand over foot as they take in worn, tired, stressed people and transform them in a fortnight into more energetic, younger looking, better functioning versions of themselves. It is a process for which you pay dearly at health farms, clinics and spas, but one which continues to attract those who can afford it because it brings such wonderful results. We've discovered that you can get the same well-proven benefits from a high-raw diet at home right now – *without* paying a fortune – by using the foods readily available in your local shops.

The problem is, suggest to most people that they increase the quantity of uncooked foods in their diet, and they feel quite confused. 'But how?' they ask. 'I can't go on eating salads all the time, can I?' The answer is simple – of course not. *Certainly not*, if you mean by salads the usual limp lettuce leaf with its familiar slice of tomato, cucumber and half a boiled egg. But, as we hope to show you in this book, the range of foods available to create Raw Energy Cuisine is enormous – a real cornucopia of delight. With them you can make beautiful hors d'oeuvres, super soups, salads which are so attractive and delicious they form the centre for a whole meal, plus a myriad of irresistible dressings, luscious drinks, sorbets and ice creams, seductive sweets, rich seed cheeses and dips, as well as breads, loaves and pâtés – a far cry from an ascetic's fare. We use such dishes to create parties which are favourites with children (and good for them too); luxurious slimmer's meals; breakfasts to keep you in top form all day long; dinners which never leave you feeling sluggish or heavy; and what we call our Fabulous Feasts where our massive round table is literally covered with nutritious pleasures for our large family and many friends.

We hope this book will give you an idea of just how simple, delicious and fun a Raw Energy way of eating can be. In it you will find all the recipes we've used in our Raw Energy television series and video, plus many more which are particular favourites with our family. We hope you will try them – and that they will help you gradually increase the number of fresh foods you eat. The recipes should be used far more as guidelines than formulae which are to be strictly followed. Our measurements are not too rigid. One of the many wonderful things about uncooked foods is that, once you get accustomed to some of the principles of Raw Energy food preparation, any recipe is little more than a suggestion offering inspiration and encouragement to create your own masterpieces.

When you do we would love to hear about them. Meantime we'd like to share with you some of our best loved recipes. We hope you'll like them!

The Raw Energy Kitchen

The mainstay of our kitchen is not the hob or the oven but our food processor. It is the one piece of equipment we would never want to do without. And because we are such a large family we have one of the big varieties which holds twice the ordinary quantity of soups, vegetables, nuts and sweets. For although most recipes in this book can be made by hand, the addition of a food processor to your kitchen equipment is such a boon in the time and energy it saves (you can prepare a whole salad meal in about five minutes), that it would be a pity to have to do without one – particularly if you are preparing food for more than two people.

A Simple Processor

There are many different models on the market, most of which we have tried, and some of which we have found completely infuriating. Processors vary enormously in the convenience of use as well as their durability. When buying a food processor it is best to choose the simplest one you can find. Those big all-purpose kitchen machines which do everything are not only a pain to put together, take apart and clean, but you are forever hunting for some little part you need for what you are doing when you could have your soup, salad or muesli finished already.

Each machine comes with several attachments. There is a blade which is excellent for grinding nuts and seeds, homogenising vegetables for soups and loaves, and making dressings, dips and sweets. The grater (some come with two – a fine and a coarse) is ideal for fruit when making muesli or for some salads, the slicer for other salads and desserts. Most food processors also have a pastry attachment – a little white plastic blade which we have always found totally useless even for making pastry. The ordinary blade does everything better.

Blender Aid

A blender too can be helpful for making energy shakes or even grinding nuts and seeds – provided you supply yourself with something like a chopstick to clear the blade when you are blending dry ingredients. If you have to choose between a blender and a processor – go for the processor, since you can do everything in it you can do in a blender. But if you are fortunate enough to have both you will probably find that the blender is easier to use for drinks while the processor works better for everything else. Even a coffee grinder can be useful for grinding small quantities of nuts if you have nothing else.

The other piece of equipment which we use often but which is by no means necessary is a centrifuge juicer for extracting vegetables juices and all fruit juices except citrus ones. We love vegetable juices – our favourite is a combination of carrot and apple which we spike with other goodies such as spinach, cabbage, berries, pineapple etc. Once you get used to the taste of fresh apple juice made this way it is like eating real Russian caviar for the first time – you never want the supermarket shelf imitation.

Hand Help

If you don't have access to this kind of electric wizardry – or even if you do – there are some useful little mechanical gadgets which can be enormously useful to the Raw Energy cook. For instance the Swiss, the French and the

Dutch have well-designed food mills for grating and chopping which you can use instead of a food processor to shred vegetables and fruits. But when buying one make sure it comes apart easily, has stainless steel blades and is simple to clean. We often use an ordinary stainless steel grater for making single bowls of muesli or for grating cheese. The reason for the stainless steel is that it does not oxidize and therefore does not destroy vitamin C in the foods you are shredding as do many of the other metals.

A Good Edge

Several sharp knives in different sizes and a couple of good chopping boards are indispensable to the Raw Energy chef. Here we break our stainless steel rule simply because you can get a much better edge on a carbon steel knife. A knife sharpener is an absolute must. So is a good vegetable brush – mark it *Vegetables* so it doesn't get used by some uninformed member of the family to scrub the wheels of his car. Another little gadget we use a lot is a salad washer – a basket in which you can spin your washed lettuce leaves to dry them before turning them into a seductive salad.

All together a Raw Energy chef needs very few utensils. You can forget the heavy pots and pans and greasy dishes which are so hard to wash up. Just for the fun of it we tend to collect different salad platters, little dishes for dressings and dips and simple one-person-meal-size bowls for dish salads which we always make sure are made from natural substances – glass, pottery, earthenware or wood rather than plastic or metal. And, of course, we always steer clear of anything made of aluminium that could come in contact with food since in the presence of acid foods such as tomatoes, aluminium, oxide tends to form which, when repeatedly taken into the body with the foods, can cause the serious symptoms of aluminium poisoning.

Finally the thing you need most, unless you are going to be cutting your lettuces from the garden, one moment and popping them into salads the next, is refrigeration. You can shop a couple of times a week provided you have a good-sized refrigerator to keep fresh things in. We even store our nuts, seeds, and oils in the fridge to protect them from oxidation. And we tend to wash many of our vegetables as soon as we get them home before putting them into vegetable bins in the refrigerator. This means that when we go down to the kitchen to prepare a luscious dish salad for lunch they are all freshly clean and waiting for us. This cuts preparation time down to between three and five minutes per salad.

Breakfasts

Breakfast quite literally means the meal at which you break your fast of the night. It needs to be light but full of the kind of energy that can sustain you through the morning without flagging. Few breakfasts can do that. Eat the standard bowl of processed dried cereal sprinkled with white sugar and you are likely to be reaching for a sticky bun by eleven 'just to see you through'. Go instead for the old-fashioned British breakfast of greasy eggs and bacon, and its high fat content can have you feeling dull-headed while the excess protein tends to make your system acid and you more prone to stress reactions as a result. Raw Energy breakfasts are different. They are fresh, fine-flavoured, sustaining and easy to prepare. They never leave you feeling heavy or over-full.

In this section we include many variations and options because we believe that there is no one 'right' breakfast dish to suit everyone. A manual labourer, for instance, will need a more calorific and sustaining meal than a person who sits behind a desk all day. Also, depending on the season, certain foods are more appropriate and more readily available. So here we suggest recipes for the old and young, for summer and winter. The important thing is to experiment to find which breakfast suits your needs best.

Note about Allergies

Many people, whether they know it or not, suffer from food allergies or sensitivities, the two most common being to milk products and wheat. Such a sensitivity can cause bloatedness, chronic fatigue, abdominal pains, skin blemishes and even depression. Many of our recipes which include either milk products or wheat have milk-free and wheat-free variations for those who prefer to avoid these products. It is sometimes worth eliminating either one or both from your diet for a week or so as an experiment to see if it makes any difference to the way you feel.

Milk is one of the most over-rated foods. It is great for calves but many people feel better without milk or milk products in their diet at all. As for wheat and its most famous ingredient bran – for some it is fine. For others that wonderful wholegrain bread or bran sprinkled on yoghurt or cereals can actually be constipating instead of laxative. There are so many other grains which are excellent sources of fibre. Oats, for example, offer a far more digestible fibre than bran and have health benefits beyond their bulking ability.

MUESLI – SWISS MAGIC

Muesli was originally the invention of the acclaimed Swiss physician Max Bircher-Benner who made it famous as part of his effective system of healing based on a high-raw diet. It, like the rest of his nutritional plan, grew out of the discovery (a discovery which at the time was no less revolutionary than it is today) that when you put sick people on a diet of all raw or mostly raw foods, they get better. For this kind of diet appears to trigger the body's own natural healing powers and encourage them to re-balance an ailing body, restore energy levels and (we have learnt to our amazement) even help stabilize a troubled mind. European experts in high-raw nutrition developed world-wide reputations for their work by curing thousands of their diverse illnesses – including the famous

Albert Schweitzer of serious diabetes, and his wife of tuberculosis (a sickness which early this century was one of our biggest killers).

Muesli was for Bircher-Benner – as it has become for us – the standard breakfast fare. And, like his original muesli, our Raw Energy breakfasts bear little resemblance to that heavy sugar-loaded dry grain variety you can buy in supermarkets these days. For real muesli is not centred on grains. It is more a fruit dish with just a hint of whole grains used as a base. Dried grains in too great a quantity cause stomach upsets for many people. But when these grains are used only in small amounts and when they have been soaked in a little water overnight their starches break down into natural sugars which are not only sweet but easy to digest. The grains in our muesli give it a sustaining quality which is sufficient for even the most physically active people.

When making muesli you can either use a food processor and do enough for the whole family at once, or with a simple hand grater make one bowl. But be sure to experiment with all the many variations depending on what kind of fruits are in season. Each has its own delicious character.

Raw Muesli

This recipe calls for an apples, but you can use almost any fruit instead, or add extra fruit in season. . . . It serves one person.

2 tbsp oatflakes (or a combination of oat, rye, wheat etc.), soaked overnight in a little water or fruit juice (e.g. pineapple), a handful of raisins (soaked), 1 apple or firm pear (grated), ½ lemon, 2 tbsp plain yoghurt, 1 tsp honey, 1 tbsp chopped nuts (e.g. almonds and Brazils), ½ tsp powdered cinnamon or ginger.

Mix together the soaked oatflakes and the raisins. Combine with this mixture a grated apple or pear with a squeeze of lemon juice and the natural plain yoghurt. Drizzle with honey and sprinkle with chopped nuts and cinnamon or ginger.

Banana Muesli Add a banana sliced in quarters lengthwise and then chopped crosswise into small pieces. Or mash a banana with a little yoghurt or fruit juice and use as a topping.

Summer Muesli Add a handful of raspberries, strawberries, blackcurrants or pitted cherries to the basic muesli, or substitute the apple for a finely diced peach or nectarine.

Winter Muesli Soak a selection of dried fruits – such as apricots, sultanas, figs, dates, pears – overnight in water. Dice into small pieces, or cut up with a pair of scissors and add to the other muesli ingredients. Spice with a pinch of nutmeg.

Dairy-Free Muesli Substitute the yoghurt for some fresh fruit juice such as apple, orange or grape. To thicken the juice, blend with a little fresh fruit such as banana, pear or apple.

Blended Muesli For old people or young children it is a good idea to blend all the muesli ingredients together in a processor. This gives a nourishing and delicious purée which requires no chewing.

FRUIT

Not only are fruits some of the most delicious natural foods available, they also have remarkable properties for spring-cleaning the body and are excellent biochemical antidotes to stress.

Because fruits contain many natural acids such as citric and malic acid, they have an acid pH reaction in digestion; however, since they are also a rich source of alkaline-forming minerals, their reaction in the blood is alkaline. This reaction helps neutralize the acidic by-products of stress as well as the waste products of metabolism which are also acidic. That is why fruits are so highly prized as a means of internally cleansing the body. Many healthy people insist that a few days on fruit alone helps clear out whatever internal rubbish they need to get rid of, and leaves them looking and feeling great.

Fruit contains very little protein but it is very high in the mineral potassium which needs to be balanced with sodium for perfect health in the body. Because most people in the West eat far too much sodium in the form of table salt and an excess of protein as well (which leaches important minerals from the bones and tissues), eating good quantities of fruit can help re-balance a body, improve its functioning, and make you feel more energetic as well. Fruit also contains natural sugars together with natural fibre. This combination means that your body is able to make good use of the energy such natural sugars provide without experiencing blood-sugar problems which lead to fatigue and can come from eating refined sugar. Fruit is also an important source of certain vitamins and minerals which are particularly important in protecting you from illness – especially vitamin C.

Finally, because fruits are naturally sweet and because we are born with an innate liking for sweet things, a snack of fruit or a sweet of fresh fruit after a meal can be tremendously satisfying to the palate. And there is such a variety of beautiful textures, colours and tastes to choose from – from the sensuous softness of persimmons and the super-sweetness of fresh figs, to the exhilarating crunch of the finest English apple.

SOME DELICIOUS AND NUTRITIOUS MUESLI SPRINKLES

These are 'extras' which can be placed in bowls at the breakfast table for people to help themselves to:

THREE-SEED MIX Grind together in a blender or processor 1C each of sesame, sunflower and pumpkin seeds. (Grind the sesame seeds first on their own very well until their husks are broken down, then add the other seeds and blend.) Keep the mixture in an airtight jar in the fridge and use to sprinkle on mueslis or salads. The three seeds together make an excellent complement of protein and essential fatty acids.

COCONUT One of our favourite sprinkles is dried coconut flakes toasted lightly under the grill until golden brown. You can mix the coconut with sesame seeds and toast together for a tasty and nutritious sprinkle.

WHEATGERM This, too, is delicious toasted. Sprinkle a tablespoon over a bowl of muesli for added vitamins B and E.

MOLASSES If you can find unsulphured molasses it makes a wonderful vitamin-and-mineral-rich sweetener to replace honey for muesli. But beware of sulphured molasses – it tastes revolting!

NUTS A few toasted whole nuts such as hazels make a nice crunchy addition to a creamy muesli.

LECITHIN Especially good for slimmers, a little lecithin sprinkled into a bowl of muesli may help emulsify the fats in the body and provides several important nutrients. For Slimmer's Porridge, see page 391.

ENERGY SHAKES

One of our favourite breakfasts is a Raw Energy shake. You simply put all the ingredients you want into a blender or food processor and whip them up in seconds to give a sustaining instant drink. One of us, Susannah, does a lot of dancing and running, and finds that an energy shake, which is easy to digest and packed with goodness, is the ideal breakfast for instant and sustained energy.

Yohurt Shake

1C plain yoghurt, 1 ripe banana, a few drops vanilla essence, 1 tsp honey, 1 tsp coconut (optional)

Combine the ingredients thoroughly in a blender. As a variation try replacing the banana with a handful of berries, half a papaya or mango, or a few chunks of fresh pineapple.

Nut-Milk Shake

This is the dairy-free alternative to the first shake. For extra goodness add a teaspoon of brewer's yeast (the de-bittered kind is the most bearable), a tablespoon of wheatgerm, or the yolk of an egg, and blend well.

⅓C almonds (blanched), ⅔C water, 5 pitted dates, few drops of vanilla essence, 1 tsp honey

Blend the almonds and the water really well until the mixture is smooth. You can use unblanched almonds and strain the mixture at this point to remove the ground-up husks. Add the other ingredients and process well. Serve immediately.

Apricot Shake Use apricots, fresh or dried, instead of the dates and add a handful of sunflower seeds to the nuts before you blend.

Grape Shake Use fruit juice such as grape (or apple) instead of the water, and raisins instead of the dates. Omit the honey and vanilla if desired.

You can make the yoghurt drink with milk for a thinner beverage – soya milk is nice.

If you are using yoghurt, why not try making your own? It's very simple and doesn't require a lot of expensive equipment. The easiest way to make it is in a wide-mouthed flask, but an earthenware crock or dish kept in a warm place will do just as well. We use two methods – the traditional one where you warm your milk to blood heat, and a simplified method that calls for warm water and powdered skimmed milk.

Home-Made Yoghurt

We prefer goat's milk to cow's because it is richer in vitamins and minerals, and because its fats are emulsified which makes it easier to digest. In fact, many people who are allergic to cow's milk can take goat's or sheep's milk quite comfortably.

2 pints (about a litre) milk (preferably goat's or sheep's), 2 heaped tbsp plain natural yoghurt (starter)

Warm milk in a saucepan to just above blood heat (test it as you would a baby's bottle). Pour into a flask or crock and add 2 heaped tablespoons of plain natural yoghurt. This can be cow's or goat's yoghurt, but it is important that it is *live yoghurt*, and that it doesn't have any fruit or sugar in it. Read the label to be sure that it contains a real yoghurt culture which is needed to transform the milk.

Stir the starter in well and replace the lid of the thermos flask. If you are using a non-insulated container, wrap it in a blanket and place it in an airing cupboard or on top of a radiator. If you have an Aga or Rayburn, place the dish on a wire cooling tray on top of it. Otherwise you can heat an oven for ten minutes as hot as it can go and then switch it off. Put the container inside and leave it, without opening the door, overnight. After 6–8 hours you will have cultured the yoghurt.

Transfer it to the fridge and use it for muesli, drinks, soups, dressings, frozen desserts etc. You can then use this yoghurt as the starter for your next batch and go on indefinitely. If your yoghurt goes sour, you'll have to buy another starter and begin afresh.

Instant Low-Fat Yoghurt

One of the very simplest methods for making yoghurt is to use low-fat milk powder. Make up two pints (about a litre) of milk in a blender, using one and a half times the amount of powdered milk suggested on the packet. If you use boiling water from a kettle and add cold water to it you can get just the temperature of milk you need and don't have to bother heating your milk in a saucepan. Add the two tablespoons of plain yoghurt as in the ordinary method and leave in a suitable container for about eight hours. If you want a really thick yoghurt, e.g. for dips, simply add more skimmed milk powder when you make up the milk.

COFFEE

For many people the focus of breakfast is a cup of coffee – or several. They rely on coffee to give them the pick-me-up they need to get themselves off to work. The problem with coffee is that its stimulating benefits are short-lived, so that by the time eleven o'clock comes around you find you need another cup to keep you going and by the end of the day you have consumed half a dozen cupfuls and still feel exhausted. For this reason the Raw Energy breakfast eliminates coffee altogether. The kinds of fresh energy-rich foods contained in our mueslis and shakes will give you the *sustained* energy you need.

Coffee also robs your body of many valuable minerals necessary for optimal health. If you like a warm drink it is far better to try one of the cereal beverages made of chicory and barley sweetened with a little honey or molasses. Or try a herb tea blend – see the section on herb teas on page 400 for suggestions.

Lunches

The ideal Raw Energy lunch is a splendid dish salad filled with different vegetables, fruits, sprouted seeds, dips and seed and nut cheeses. We prepare one of these salads for each member of the family in large individual dishes in a matter of minutes. And because each person has his own salad, if there is one particular vegetable he doesn't like – onions, say – it can be left out very easily.

Each time we make a dish salad the ingredients vary depending on what we have available. We are always experimenting with new ways of chopping and combining vegetables, fruits etc. We also grow our own sprouted seeds and beans and then keep them in the fridge in polythene bags to sprinkle over salads. Seed and nut cheeses make a delicious but rich contribution to such a salad. We sometimes spoon a little straight into the dish salad or spread some on to pumpernickel bread, rye crackers or oatcakes to eat with it. The dressings we use for dish salads are what we call dip-dressings. They are thick dressings which can be used as dips to dunk crudités into, or thinned a little with water or juice to pour over vegetables. Finally we often toast a few seeds – pumpkins, sunflower or sesame – to sprinkle over the top of the salad.

Dish salads vary from the elaborate to the very simple: for example a selection of fresh greens – lettuces and herbs straight from the garden – torn into bite-sized pieces, tossed with a handful of chopped spring onions and topped with a tofu or hummus dressing. Here are a few examples to give the general idea. After that it's up to you to improvise and make up your own combinations with whatever you like best. (As you will see, we deliberately haven't specified quantities.)

354

Dish Salad 1

Make a base of radicchio leaves (or any other lettuce) to line the dish. Then arrange in segments:

grated carrot placed inside a ring of red pepper and topped with a few fresh garden peas

a small bunch of watercress inside a ring of sweet yellow pepper

half an avocado (brush with lemon juice or olive oil to prevent it going brown) filled with radish slices

a handful of Chinese bean sprouts (mung)

a few diagonal slices of cucumber

a few cauliflower and broccoli florets

some grated raw beetroot

some grated white radish

mustard and cress

a tomato sliced into segments – but not all the way through – so that it looks like flower petals.

Dish Salad 2

Line bowl with chopped Chinese leaves, then arrange the following:

celery and carrot sticks looped through rings of sweet peppers

a few slices of fennel

a few slices of baby turnip (raw)

some mangetout (topped and tailed)

some slices of apple

slices of red onion

radish roses (made from cutting zig-zags around the middle of the radish and separating two halves)

a small bunch of grapes

watercress and parsley

an orange sliced in segments with the skin left on for decoration, but peeled back in sections so that it can easily be removed

a handful of chickpea sprouts

Dish Salad 3

Make a base with alfalfa sprouts, then:

arrange around the dish grated carrot, red cabbage, white cabbage and beetroot
add sliced mushrooms, black olives and spring onions
sprinkle raisins over the grated vegetables and add a spoonful of seed and nut cheese (see page 360)

Dish Salad 4

Make a base by shredding tender spinach leaves finely (remove the stalks), then arrange around the dish:

a handful of baby button mushrooms with their stems trimmed
half an avocado, diced (simply slice the flesh in its shell several times first vertically and then horizontally, then scoop out the avocado with a spoon)
some diced red pepper
apple rings (remove the core from the apple and slice crosswise)
thin slices of Jerusalem artichoke, kohlrabi or new potatoes (raw)
toasted pumpkin seeds

Dish Salad 5

Use shredded iceberg lettuce as a base, then arrange:

thin slices of carrot and courgette (the slicer attachment on a food processor is ideal for this)
a few cherry tomatoes
sweetcorn (raw, scraped off the cob, or cooked on the cob)
a few toasted hazelnuts
mustard and cress

The appearance of a dish salad is very important. Fortunately the brilliant colours of fresh vegetables and fruit are quite stunning. It is nice to experiment with different decorative ways of chopping fruits and vegetables to make attractive garnishes.

DIP-DRESSINGS

Here are some of our favourite dip-dressings. We particularly like them with dish salads because of their lovely textures, but of course you can use a regular vinaigrette or mayonnaise-type dressing instead. (For more dressing suggestions see pages 372–75)

Curried Avocado

Even those who say they don't like avocados adore this one!

1–2 avocados, 1C (more or less, to give the desired consistency) fresh orange juice, 1 tsp curry powder, 2 tsp vegetable bouillon powder, fresh herbs (e.g. lovage and French parsley), 1 small clove garlic (optional)

Peel and stone the avocado(s). Blend all the ingredients together in a food processor until smooth.

Raw Hummus

1C chickpea sprouts (about 1 inch or 2 cm long), juice of 1 lemon, a little orange juice to thin, 1 clove garlic, vegetable bouillon powder, 2 tbsp tahini, chives or spring onions, paprika

Blend the chickpea sprouts very finely in the food processor. Add lemon and orange juices, garlic, bouillon powder and tahini, and blend well. Spoon into a bowl and top with chopped chives or spring onions, and paprika.

357

Tofu Dip

1C tofu, juice of 1 lemon, 1 tsp wholegrain Meaux mustard, vegetable bouillon powder, fresh basil and mint

Combine all the ingredients well in the food processor.

Creamed Carrot

1–2 carrots (roughly chopped), 1C tofu or cream/cottage cheese, ¼C walnuts, a handful of fresh parsley, pinch nutmeg, vegetable bouillon powder, a little water or carrot juice to thin, a few slivers of carrot to garnish

Blend the carrots well in the processor along with the tofu or cheese and nuts. Add the herbs and seasonings and a little water or juice to thin if desired. Serve in a bowl sprinkled with carrot slivers.

Ginger Dressing

1C tofu, juice of 1 lemon, 1 tsp grated lemon rind, 1 tsp honey, 1 tsp freshly grated ginger root, 1 clove garlic (pressed), 1 tbsp red wine

Blend all the ingredients together well in the food processor.

Yoghurt-Cucumber

½ cucumber, 1C thick yoghurt, 1 tbsp vinegar, 1 tsp honey, 1 tsp crushed dill and coriander, handful of walnuts, vegetable bouillon powder, garlic (optional), fresh mint

Peel the cucumber (the skin tends to make the dressing bitter) and chop roughly. Put in the processor with the other ingredients (except mint) and blend well. Serve chilled decorated with mint sprigs.

Dracula's Delight

1 small beetroot, 1C toasted or raw sunflower seeds, 2 lemons, 2 tbsp tamari, cayenne, thyme, vegetable bouillon powder, a little water to give desired consistency

Scrub and grate the beetroot. Combine in the processor with the other ingredients plus 1 teaspoon grated lemon rind. Blend well and adjust the seasoning to taste.

Tomato Treat

4–5 large tomatoes, ½C almonds, 1 tbsp tahini, juice of 1 lemon, 2 spring onions (chopped), handful of fresh basil leaves, tarragon, freshly ground black pepper, vegetable bouillon powder

Blanch the tomatoes by dropping them in boiling water for a few moments, then remove the skins. Grind the almonds in the food processor and add the tomatoes and other ingredients. Save a few spring onion bits to sprinkle over the top of the dressing. Blend the mixture thoroughly and thin with a little water if necessary.

Creamy Mushroom

¼C cashew nuts, 1C mushrooms (washed and trimmed), ¼C water, 1 tbsp Minced onion, 1 tsp Meaux mustard, 1 tsp tamari, ground black pepper, parsley

Grind the nuts first in the food processor. Then add all the other ingredients (except parsley) and blend thoroughly. Garnish with fresh parsley.

Island Dip

1C egg mayonnaise (see page 373), 1 tbsp Whole Earth Tomato Ketchup, 1 tsp Meaux mustard, 2 hard-boiled eggs, a few olives, slices of red pepper or raw beetroot, fresh parsley

Combine the mayonnaise, ketchup and mustard. Chop the eggs finely – the small grater attachment on a food processor is ideal. Pit and chop the olives and finely chop the red pepper or beetroot, and parsley. Combine all the ingredients well and thin with a little water if necessary.

SEED AND NUT CHEESES

These are called cheeses because, just like dairy cheeses, they undergo the process of fermentation where some of the protein they contain is partially digested by bacteria. These cheeses are made from ground seeds and nuts. The basic recipe is very simple. Once you have made the cheese base you can add whatever seasoning and spices you wish. You then let it sit for about eight hours (or overnight) in a warm place to ferment. You can also eat seed cheeses freshly made if you prefer.

Basic Seed and Nut Cheese

1C nuts (e.g. cashews, almonds, pecans), 1C seeds (sunflower, pumpkin), ¾–1C water, 1 tsp vegetable bouillon powder

Blend the nuts and seeds finely in a food processor. Add the water and bouillon powder and blend to give a firm paste. (At this point we usually divide the mixture into two parts and season each differently. Choose seasonings from the list below). Combine bases well with the seasonings. Turn into dishes. Leave covered with a tea towel for several hours. Refrigerate and use to spread on vegetable and fruit slices – e.g. apples, cucumbers, carrots, lettuce leaves – or spread thinly on crackers.

Sage and Onion Add 3 spring onions or a little minced red onion, 6 sage leaves (or 1 tsp dried) and 2 tbsp wine to the basic recipe and garnish with a little chopped onion.

Garlic and Herb Add 2 tbsp mixed fresh (or 2 tsp dried) herbs – e.g. parsley and oregano – 1 clove garlic and juice of ½ lemon.

Nutmeg Add ½ tsp freshly ground nutmeg and 1 tsp tahini.

Curry Add 1 tsp curry powder and a squeeze of lemon juice.

Caraway Add 2 tsp toasted seeds to the base.

We often eat oatcakes or rye crackers with lunch and have a glass of vegetable or fruit juice or mineral water. Sometimes we like to eat our own home-made crackers which are raw and have to be made ahead of time to dry and crisp up. One of our favourites is Sunflower Wafers which can be made savoury or sweet and make great snacks at any time during the day.

Savoury Sunflower Wafers

2 tbsp sesame seeds (toasted if you prefer), 1C sunflower seeds, 1 tbsp tamari, 2 tbsp water, few chopped chives

Grind the sesame seeds finely in the food processor. Add the remaining ingredients and grind well. The mixture should be of a stiff dough consistency. Pinch off small pieces and roll into balls. Flatten down on a board with the palm of your hand and then use a fish slice to lift off. Place on a wire cooling tray and leave in a warm place or in the sun to dry out.

Sweet Sunflower Wafers

Follow the same instructions as above but using the following ingredients.

1C sunflower seeds, ¼ C raisins or sultanas, ½ tsp cinnamon or allspice, 2 tbsp water

Supersalads

A Supersalad is the focus of the main meal of the day whether it be lunch or dinner. The salad is given the position of honour and the meat, fish, chicken, game, eggs or grain assume the normal position of the 'side salad'. In this way 50 to 75 per cent of the meal is raw. The 'side' dishes can be served in a separate bowl next to the salad or combined with the salad. For example, we often toss chopped hard-boiled egg into a salad, lay slivers of roasted chicken breast on top of a salad or make a vegetable salad with a base of cold cooked rice, millet or buckwheat. Then there are the dressings which range from egg and tahini mayonnaises to French and seed and nut dressings. To finish off the Supersalad we prepare a range of delicious salad sprinkles to dredge over the top.

In this section you will find major and minor salads. The major salads are substantial meal in themselves. The minor salads can be served with other dishes, for example with fish, poultry or game, lentil stews or grain dishes as brown rice, or several of them can be made and served together as separate courses to make up a main meal. Either way you'll find salad recipes for all year round as well as some unusual and exciting taste combinations.

MAJOR SALADS

Garden Crunch

We like to use purple sprouting broccoli from the garden in this, but the ordinary green variety, or a mixture of both, is just as good.

½ iceberg lettuce, 2 or 3 broccoli stalks (use the stems as well as the tops), 1C finely shredded red cabbage, 2–3 tomatoes, several mushrooms, handful of fresh garden peas, 1 shallot or small red onion, a handful of toasted pumpkin seeds

Shred the lettuce and place in a bowl. Add the broccoli tops broken into small pieces, and the stems peeled and sliced crosswise. Shred the red cabbage really finely, chop the tomatoes and slice the mushrooms. Add the peas and the shallot or onion cut into rings. Toss all the ingredients together and top with toasted pumpkin seeds. Serve with a thinned mayonnaise dressing.

Summer Symphony

This salad is a play on colours and shapes – the more variety, and the more you grow yourself, the better.

1 small head of lettuce (Cos is good), 1C small cauliflower florets, 2 celery stalks (finely chopped first lengthwise, then crosswise), 2 carrots (coarsely grated or cut into matchsticks), 6 whole cherry tomatoes, 4 sliced radishes, 1 green pepper cut into thin strips, a few leaves of watercress, sweetcorn off the cob or alfalfa sprouts to garnish

Place the lettuce leaves, torn into bite-sized pieces or shredded, into a bowl – a clear glass bowl is nice for this one as you can see all the beautiful colours through it. Prepare the vegetables and arrange in layers in the bowl. Dress with a thinned mayonnaise dressing, perhaps blended with a tomato or two, and top with sweetcorn or alfalfa sprouts. You can lay slivers of chicken breast on the top and sprinkle with paprika.

Spun Spinach Salad

Many people grow spinach in their gardens and don't know what to do with it. This salad really makes the most of it. You can use any greens instead of spinach, such as perpetual beet or even lettuce. Try to choose the young leaves as they are more tender and sweet. Save the older ones for cooking.

A large bunch of spinach leaves (stems removed), 3 spring onions, 2 handfuls of button mushrooms (finely sliced), a few red radishes (sliced), a handful of toasted cashews or sunflower seeds, 3 hard-boiled eggs

The trick here is to make the spinach look spun. Use a very sharp knife and hold the bunched together leaves tightly in one hand. Cut them as finely as possible as if you were cutting wafer-thin slices of bread. The result will be long thin green strips which look and taste delicious. Chop the spring onions finely so that their taste blends with the spinach and add the other ingredients. The mushrooms should be sliced crosswise – leaving the stems on and just trimming the ends if they look tatty. Peel the hard-boiled eggs and chop or grate into the salad. Toss with a French dressing with garlic.

Italian Salad

The Italians make some of the most delicious salads of all because they grow such splendid vegetables. When we visit Italy we buy several packets of seeds to grow different types of lettuces and basil in our own garden.

1 Italian red lettuce (radicchio) and 1 small Cos lettuce (both finely shredded), 1 red and 1 yellow sweet pepper cut into rings, 1–2 large Italian tomatoes (sliced), 4 radishes (cut into segments), 1 red onion (cut into thin rings), a few thinly sliced button mushrooms, fennel seeds, sliced Mozzarella cheese (optional)

Make a nest of the two shredded lettuces in a shallow dish and arrange the other vegetables in the centre, sprinkling the onion and mushroom slices in last. Toss with a spicy Italian dressing with lots of fresh basil, and sprinkle with toasted fennel seeds, sliced cheese, and freshly ground black pepper if desired.

Jungle Slaw

2C white cabbage (shredded or finely grated), a handful of tender green beans (raw or steamed, cut into slivers diagonally), 2 carrots (grated), ½ onion (grated), ½ red or yellow pepper (chopped into very small pieces), 1C unsalted peanuts (toasted under the grill until golden)

Combine all the ingredients except the peanuts. Make a dressing with peanut oil (if possible) and orange juice (see Citrus French dressing for a guideline, page 379). You can add a little chopped chilli pepper if you're adventurous. Add the peanuts at the last minute so that they don't become soggy.

Sunshine Salad

We often add fresh or dried fruits to savoury salads for a delightful flavour contrast. Fresh pineapple is wonderful. It contains an enzyme, bromelain, which helps digest protein. Make sure it is ripe by pulling out one of its centre leaves. If it comes out quite easily, then it is ready to use.

A few leaves of crisp lettuce, 1 medium-sized fresh pineapple, 2 coarsely grated carrots, 2 finely chopped sticks of celery, 2 handfuls of sultanas (or raisins) soaked in water for a few hours to plump them up if possible, ½ tsp celery seeds, 1 tsp dry mustard mixed with mayonnaise for dressing, wheat sprout roasts (see Sprinkles, page 371).

Wash then crisp the lettuce leaves in the fridge. Peel the pineapple – it isn't necessary to core it – and dice it into fairly small cubes. Prepare the carrots and celery. Combine these with the pineapple and add with the sultanas. Sprinkle with celery seeds and serve on a bed of crisp lettuce leaves with a light mayonnaise or French dressing. Sprinkle finely with wheat sprout roasts.

High-Fibre Salad

This salad is made with a base of rice, millet or buckwheat which has been cooked and then cooled. The grains make a filling salad while supplying plenty of good-quality fibre.

2 sticks celery, 2 tomatoes, ½ red pepper, 3C cooked brown rice, millet or buckwheat, handful of walnuts, 2 spring onions

Finely dice the celery, carrot, tomatoes and red pepper. Stir into the grain with a handful of walnuts. Top with chopped spring onions and dress with a French dressing with lots of fresh parsley.

VEGETABLES

Fresh raw vegetables are surely the most neglected of all foods for health. Our consumption of these live foods has decreased dramatically in the last fifty years as a result of sophisticated food processing and changes in dietary habits. When grown on healthy soil and carefully prepared, these humble yet beautiful products of the earth are not only irresistibly delicious, they are also potent protectors against premature ageing and the degenerative illnesses which plague Western civilisation in the twentieth century. In clinical studies and laboratory experiments raw vegetables and fruits have been shown to protect against cancer in animals, to lower cholesterol levels in the blood, and to increase stamina and endurance.

Many people avoid fresh vegetables believing that they are not really the important foods because they don't contain protein – so they fill themselves with cooked foods, meat, eggs and milk products instead. In fact cooking changes the biochemical structure of amino acids – the building blocks of proteins – and fatty acids, and makes them only partly digestible. At the world-famous Max Planck Institute for Nutritional Research in Germany, scientists have shown that you need only half the amount of protein in your diet if you eat protein foods raw instead of cooked. Some green vegetables contain proteins of the highest quality. Eaten together with wholegrain bread and legumes or pulses they provide the best quality protein you will find anywhere without the added fat you get from meat. For instance a green salad has a very high protein value in proportion to its calories. And vegetable protein has another important advantage as well: unlike meat or milk products, it does not come with lots of fat attached. Finally, fresh raw vegetables are high in natural unadulterated fibre.

The best vegetables are those you grow yourself organically. If you are lucky enough to have a garden – even a small one – save all the uncooked leftovers and turn them into compost for fertilizer. Even in winter you can grow some delicious salads and root vegetables in a greenhouse of under cloches. The quality of organic produce is far superior to chemically fertilized fruits and vegetables – not to mention all of the vitamins which are lost in foods when they are picked, stored, shipped and sit on shop shelves. We go to the garden to pick our vegetables and fifteen minutes later they are gracing our dinner table in salad bowls. That is the best way to preserve their nutritional value as well as to experience the fullness of their flavour. If you are a flat dweller without a garden you can sprout fresh seeds and grains in jars or trays on your windowsill (see page 383).

How you treat your vegetables once you cut them or buy them from the shops also determines a lot how they taste, and how much of their energy-enhancing goodness you preserve. Scrub anything that will stand up to a good scrubbing, using a brush marked *Veg Only*. Scrubbing vegetables is better than peeling since many of the valuable vitamins and minerals are stored directly beneath their skins. Never soak vegetables for long periods. They are better washed briefly under running water so you don't allow water-soluble vitamins to leach out of them. Always keep vegetables as cool as possible (even carrots and turnips are best kept in the refrigerator), and use them as soon as you can. When shopping for fresh things be demanding – choose your own cauliflower and make sure it is a good one. Don't be intimidated by pushy greengrocers who want to pass off on you the leftovers before they bring their new stock in. Demand the best and you will get it. Your palate and your health will be grateful that you do.

MINOR SALADS

These are some of the very simple lighter salads. You can serve several together as a full meal or use one instead of having cooked vegetables with your meat, fish etc.

Wild Gypsy Salad

Most people groan at the thought of a green salad – envisaging wilted rubbery lettuce leaves with a piece of floppy cucumber. For us green salad is one of the greatest raw food delights. We grow all sorts of lettuces and greens in our garden and toss them together with our favourite herbs to make this simple but seductive salad.

There is no precise recipe for it, as each time we make it it turns out a little different.

Gather a few of the following: Cos lettuce, butterhead, sugarloaf, radicchio, iceberg, curly endive, dandelion leaves, sorrel, chard, purslane, chickweed, lamb's lettuce, corn salad, land and garden cress, mustard and cress, salad rape, tarragon, parsley, nasturtium, chervil, basil, lovage, lemon balm and marjoram.

Rinse the leaves and herbs and spin dry. Place in a tied polythene bag in the fridge for a few minutes to crisp up. Tear the leaves into bite-sized pieces and toss into a bowl. Add some finely chopped chives or spring onions if desired. You can also add a couple of tablespoons of toasted sesame seeds or some sliced radishes. (See Salad Sprinkles page 371, for more ideas.) Dress with a citrus or mustardy French dressing and serve at once.

Winter Chunk Salad

Slaws are ideal winter salads because in the cold months when lettuce is hard to come by cabbage is a staple. Another perfect ingredient for the winter season is sprouted seeds and beans which can be grown anytime anywhere (see sprouting instructions, pages 383–6). To make this salad you simply combine whatever winter vegetables and sprouts you have available and toss them together with a creamy mayonnaise dressing.

Select three of the following and grate: carrots, turnip, Jerusalem artichokes, kohlrabi, white radish, beetroot. Add a handful of mixed sprouts – e.g. mung, lentil, wheat, alfalfa, fenugreek or chickpea. Combine with a handful of raisins and toss with a mayonnaise dressing spiced with nutmeg.

Avocado Citrus Salad

2–3 avocados, 2 oranges (or 1 grapefruit or 3 satsumas), curly endive, watercress, alfalfa sprouts, paprika

Peel and stone the avocados. Cut in slices lengthwise. Peel and slice the citrus fruit and halve the slices. Make a bed of curly endive on a large plate and lay alternating slices of avocado and citrus fruit on it. Garnish with watercress and alfalfa and dust with paprika. Serve with a citrus French dressing (see page 379).

Crisp Carrot Salad

6–8 fresh carrots, 3 spring onions, mustard and cress, juice of 1 lemon and 1 orange, 1 tsp wholegrain mustard, 2 tsp honey, ½ tsp vegetable bouillon powder, 3 tbsp olive oil, 1 tbsp fresh chopped parsley, freshly ground black pepper

Scrub the carrots well and top and tail. Slice very finely crosswise, if possible with the slicer attachment of a food processor. Finely chop the spring onions and add to the carrots along with the mustard and cress. Combine the remaining ingredients and pour over the salad. Toss well.

Bulgar Salad

3C wheat sprouts, 3 tomatoes, 2 spring onions, handful of black olives, alfalfa sprouts, parsley and mint

Lay the wheat sprouts in a flat dish. Slice the tomatoes and spring onions and place in a layer on top of the wheat. Add the olives and sprinkle with alfalfa sprouts, fresh parsley and mint. Serve with a lemon and olive oil dressing.

Apple Ginger Salad

Another very simple salad that goes with almost any dish. The ginger is a natural digest-aid.

6 green apples (Granny Smiths are best), ¼C fresh orange
juice, 1 tsp fresh grated ginger, 2 tsp clear honey, 3 tbsp
toasted sesame seeds

Quarter the apples, remove the cores and then finely slice
by hand or in a processor. Combine the orange juice,
ginger and honey, and pour over the apples immediately
to prevent them going brown. Add the toasted sesame
seeds and toss well.

SPRINKLES

Whatever your salad, whether a full mixed salad or a
simple lettuce salad, it can almost certainly be improved
by salad sprinkles. These can be put on to the top of the
salad or placed on the table in small dishes for people to
help themselves.

THE THREE SEEDS
Any or all of them – sunflower, pumpkin and sesame –
straight, ground or toasted.

OTHER SEEDS
Fennel, celery, poppy, caraway, dill, cumin (plain or
toasted).

MUSTARD AND CRESS

MINCED NUTS

FRESH HERBS
Parsley, basil, marjoram, mint, fennel, lovage, thyme,
tarragon, savory, lemon balm.

SPROUTED SEEDS AND PULSES
See page 383.

SEAWEED
Nori – a type of seaweed which is dried and pressed into
thin sheets. Delicious toasted and crumbled on to a salad.

FLOWER PETALS
Such as marigolds, nasturtiums, roses.

SOYA NUTS
These are wonderful! You simply bake soya sprouts (sprinkled with garlic powder or vegetable bouillon powder) in a moderate oven for about 15 minutes, or until brown and crunchy.

WHEAT AND BARLEY ROASTS
These have a lovely sweet flavour. Bake wheat and/or barley sprouts on a baking sheet as for soya nuts.

HARD-BOILED EGGS
Particularly attractive if you separate the yolk and white once boiled, and grate, then sprinkle in strips of white and yellow over a salad.

CHICKPEAS
Cooked and cooled then tossed into a slaw or leafy salad.

ARTICHOKE HEARTS
One exception to the 'no tinned food' general rule because they are *so* delicious.

FINELY GRATED BEETROOT
Adds colour to bland-looking salads.

GRATED HARD CHEESE

TOFU SLICES

SLICES OR STRIPS OF COLD BAKED POTATO

COLOURED POWDERS
Paprika, cayenne and cumin are nice dusted over pale vegetables and dressings to brighten them up.

SUPER DRESSINGS

Far too many people tend to rely on bottled salad-cream type dressings which are not only full of chemical additives, sugar and saturated fats, but which completely obliterate all the subtle flavours of a good salad. We always make our own salad dressings, whether they be vinaigrettes or mayonnaises, and keep them in airtight jars in the fridge to use over several days. That way you can be sure to use the best, freshest oils and you can experiment with wonderful herbs and spices to get a range of different flavours. In this section there are three main types of dressings: mayonnaises (egg and tahini based), oil/French, and seed/nut dressings. Try making one salad and dressing it two ways – you'll be surprised at what variety you can get by simply changing the dressing.

EGG MAYONNAISES

Mayonnaises are best for coleslaws, sprout, and finely chopped mixed vegetable salads. They are thick and creamy and so give body to a salad. Alternatively they can be diluted with a little water and served over a leafy salad.

Egg Mayonnaise Dressing

There seems to be some myth behind mayonnaise making and some people sweat that they can never get their mayonnaise to 'take'. It really is perfectly simple, particularly with the use of an electric blender or food processor. We have tried several ways of preparing a basic mayonnaise, and we find this one works best.

2 egg yolks, 2 tbsp cider vinegar or lemon juice, 1 tsp mustard powder or fresh French mustard, 1 tsp honey, pinch of pepper and vegetable bouillon powder, 10fl. oz or 300 ml of oil. (Olive oil makes a rather strong tasting mayonnaise and we sometimes prefer to use a lighter oil such as cold-pressed walnut or soya.)

Put all the ingredients except the oil into the blender and process at top speed for about 45 seconds, then slowly trickle the oil in through the hole in the top of the blender in a thin continuous stream. This method really does work. One reason is probably that to make a successful mayonnaise you need your ingredients to be at room temperature, and by pre-blending you warm them all (especially if you are using refrigerated eggs).

This recipe makes about a cupful of mayonnaise. It should be refrigerated in an airtight jar to cool and then eaten within a day or two. (Bought mayonnaise only keeps so well because it is loaded with preservatives.)

Once you have your basic mayonnaise you can branch out with lots of interesting flavours and spices. Here are a few suggestions:

Green Mayonnaise Add a small handful of your favourite fresh herbs, finely chopped or about a tablespoon of dried herbs such as parsley, oregano, thyme, dill, sorrel . . .

Garlic Mayonnaise Add a small crushed clove of garlic to the base.

Curry Mayonnaise Add a ½ tsp of curry powder and a dash of nutmeg.

Horseradish Mayonnaise Add 1 tsp finely grated horseradish.

Hot Mayonnaise Add a dash of Tabasco sauce.

Tomato Mayonnaise Add 2 tbsp Whole Earth Tomato Ketchup.

Paprika Mayonnaise Add 1 tsp paprika. 1t gives an attractive colour.

Mint Mayonnaise Add a handful of clean, destalked fresh mint leaves and blend.

Cheese and Onion Mayonnaise Add a little grated Parmesan or hard Cheddar and some very finely grated onion, chopped spring onions or chopped chives.

TAHINI MAYONNAISES

Basic Tahini Mayonnaise

½C tahini, juice of 1 large lemon, ½C water (or more)

Combine the tahini and lemon juice in the blender at medium speed. Add the water a little at a time to get the consistency you want.

You should keep the mayonnaise in an airtight jar and use it preferably the day you make it, but within 5 days at the most.

Plain tahini mayonnaise is a little bland on its own, but some delicious variations can be made.

Small Seed Tahini Mayonnaise Add either caraway *or* dill seeds, 1 tbsp cider vinegar, some finely grated lemon rind, a little honey and some finely grated onion if desired. You can sprinkle a few whole sesame or poppy seeds into the dressing just before you serve it.

Mexican Pepper Mayonnaise Add 2 tbsp finely chopped red and/or green sweet pepper, 1 tbsp finely minced onion, a pinch of cayenne pepper, a little mustard and ¼ tsp vegetable bouillon powder.

Herbal Mayonnaise Add ½–1 clove garlic (crushed), fresh herbs if possible (chives, basil, chervil, parsley, lovage, rosemary, finely chopped), 1 tsp vinegar and 1 tsp honey.

HERBS

The magicians of Raw Energy food preparation, fresh herbs can transform a humble salad into a Pasha's delight. We use them constantly, lavishly, and occasionally with utter abandon – when we add as many as seven different leafy herbs to a simple green salad, becoming more of a herb salad than a green salad by the time we're finished. We never add salt to any of our dishes but when you rely on herb magic to garnish your salads, seed and nut cheeses, soups and hors d'oeuvres, even the most addicted salt user will find he hardly misses the stuff.

Most of our herbs we grow in the garden because there is something about freshness which you just can't recapture from the dried varieties. And with fresh herbs you needn't worry much about choosing the wrong ones. Some of our favourites for salads include lovage (which we also use to season many salad dressings), basil, dill, the mints, sweet cicely, winter savory, fennel, chives and the parsleys. In the summer we cull them from the garden. Some we dry by hanging from beams in our kitchen for a few days and then store them in airtight jars for winter use. Others – the more succulent herbs such as parsley, basil, and chives – can be deep frozen in sprigs then simply chopped and used when needed. If you live in a flat or don't have a garden you can grow herbs in pots in the kitchen window where they lend their own beauty to the room as well as offering a constant supply of culinary delights. Thyme, marjoram and winter savory will grow beautifully in pots indoors over the winter. So will parsley. Once you begin to play about with herb magic you will probably find, as we have, that you never want to be without these lovely plants.

Here are some of the most common herbs and what we find them useful for:

BASIL We probably use this herb far too much because it is available only in the summer months and because it is simply so lovely. It has a distinctive flavour which is an ideal garnish for tomatoes or in large amounts mixed into a green salad. Use the leaves whole for the best possible flavour.

CHERVIL This herb is a cousin to parsley, with a delicate aniseed flavour. We use it lavishly in salads. It mixes particularly well with chives, tarragon and parsley.

CHIVES More beautiful in looks than in flavour, we think, chives are great for sprinkling on to sunflower wafers or in seed cheeses. We find them not strong enough for most salads and prefer instead spring onions or a little chopped shallots.

DILL It goes wonderfully with yoghurt dressings, cucumbers, and beetroot and apple salads, and has a gentle delicate flavour which reminds one of quiet afternoons under sun-shaded willows.

FENNEL A lacy aniseed-flavoured herb which grows immense in the summer (ours is over eight feet tall). It goes well with salsify salads, and with cucumbers, tomatoes and in vegetable loaves. It is also a lovely decorative herb to place around the edge of dish salads.

HORSERADISH It is the root here which is important. Hot and pungent, it gets added to our many mayonnaises and dips for extra zest, and it works well in seed cheeses too.

LOVAGE Perhaps the most underrated of the common herbs, lovage is wonderful mixed with the mints and yoghurt as the base of a herbal salad dressing which is as beautiful in colour as it is in flavour. We use lots of it also in our dish salads.

MARJORAM This herb comes in many variations – sweet marjoram, pot marjoram, winter marjoram, golden marjoram. Each is a little different. The sweet variety is lovely with plain green salads and goes well with tomatoes and Mediterranean vegetables. Oregano is a wild marjoram akin to our winter variety.

THE MINTS There are even more varieties than the marjorams – spearmint, peppermint, apple mint, pineapple mint, ginger mint, eau de cologne mint. We use spearmint and apple mint in green salads and many dressings. Pineapple mint with its splendid variegated leaves makes a wonderful garnish for fruit salads, drinks and also salad platters. Ginger mint is great (as are the others for that matter) in summer drinks, sorbets and punches.

PARSLEY This common herb comes in two main varieties – fine and broad leaf. For most raw dishes we prefer the broadleaf parsley because it is more delicate and pleasant to munch. Both have a rich 'green' flavour which works well with other herbs. It is great chopped in patties and loaves, in green salads and for dressings as well as being a lovely garnish for almost any dish.

SAGE This herb has a strong individual flavour and a particular affinity for onions. It is good in savoury nut dishes and adds flavour to seed and nut ferments.

SWEET CICELY Another aniseed-like herb which you can use as you would fennel. It is delicious in a carrot salad.

THYME It comes in many varieties, some of which are much richer in flavour than others, but all have a wonderful warming sweet flavour which enhances peppers, courgettes, and nut dishes as well as giving a unique flavour to sprout salads.

FRENCH DRESSINGS

Oil dressings are especially good for leafy salads such as lettuce and spinach. With the right seasonings, such as a tasty mustard and various herbs, they can be very flavourful and not at all the 'plain oil and vinegar dressing' most people know.

Basic French Dressing

¾C *olive, soy or walnut oil,* ¼C *lemon juice or cider vinegar, 1 tsp wholegrain mustard (French Meaux mustard is our favourite) or mustard powder, 2 tsp honey, a little vegetable bouillon powder and pepper to season, a small clove of crushed garlic (optional)*

Combine all the ingredients in a blender or simply place in a screw-top jar and shake well to mix. Some people like to thin the dressing and make it a little lighter by adding a couple of tablespoons of water.

Here are some suggestions for dressing beginning with the French dressing base:

Rich French Dressing Add 1 tbsp tamari (see page 426), 1 finely chopped spring onion and a dash of cayenne.

Wine Dressing Add 1 tbsp of red or white wine – white is good for salads containing fruit, and red for cabbage salads.

Herb Dressing Our favourite combination of herbs for dressings is: marjoram, basil, thyme and dill or lovage (about 3–4 tbsp in all of fresh, finely chopped, or 2 tsp dried).

Citrus Dressing Use ¾C sesame oil, juice of ½ lemon and 1 orange, and 1 tbsp vinegar in the above basic dressing. Add 1 tsp grated orange peel and ½ tsp grated lemon peel (scrub the fruits first!), a pinch of nutmeg and 1 tsp chervil. Put all the ingredients in the blender until smooth.

Spicy Italian Dressing Follow the basic recipe, using cider vinegar, and add a dash or red wine or tamari, 2 ripe peeled tomatoes, 1 tbsp finely chopped onion, garlic, ½ tsp oregano and basil, and some powdered bay leaf. Blend all the ingredients well.

Olive Dressing Use olive oil and lemon juice in the basic recipe. Add 4–6 pitted black olives, finely chopped, and a pinch of cayenne.

SEED AND NUT DRESSINGS

Seed and nut dressings are particularly 'warming' served over a winter salad, and used over a sprout or mixed vegetable salad will make a substantial meal. There are two types – fermented and unfermented. Fermented dressings take about six to twelve hours to culture, depending on the temperature. They have a taste all their own which is both sweet and tangy. As with most dressings you can begin with the base and then add herbs and spices to suit your taste. Nuts and seeds can be fermented separately to make sauces, but we prefer them in combination.

Sunflower/Cashew Dressing

This dressing is good served over grated root vegetables such as carrots. You can ferment it or serve it immediately.

½C cashews, ½C sunflower seeds, 1C water, 1tsp yeast extract or vegetable bouillon powder

Grind the nuts and seeds in a food processor as finely as possible. Add the water, then the yeast extract or vegetable bouillon and combine well. Put the mixture into a bowl and cover with a tea towel. Place in a warm spot for about eight hours (or overnight). After a couple of hours give the sauce a good stir. You may need to add more water to make the dressing thinner. The ferment should taste sweet and pleasant. If it tastes 'off' you have over-fermented it. If you wish you can season it lightly with a few fresh herbs before you serve it.

Sun-Sesame Seeds Dressing

¼C sesame seeds, ½C sunflower seeds (soaked overnight in water), 1–2 carrots, juice 1 lemon, 1 tsp honey, parsley, vegetable bouillon to taste, water

Process the sesame seeds finely in the food processor, then add the sunflower seeds and re-process. (The sesame seeds tend not to get ground up unless they are done by themselves.) Add the roughly chopped carrot(s), the lemon juice, honey and seasonings. Blend well. Add water to give the desired consistency. You can use this one right away.

Italian Pesto

A delicious sauce, particularly good served over alfalfa sprouts or a simple lettuce salad.

Ideally use 1C of pine kernels (pignoli nuts) or pistachios (if you can't get these, or they are too expensive, you can substitute almonds or pecans), ½C olive oil, 1 handful of fresh basil leaves plus a little parsley or oregano, ½ clove crushed garlic, a little grated Parmesan or Sardo cheese (if desired)

Blend or process the nuts and gradually add the oil. Add the herbs (remove the stalks and use only the leaves) and garlic, then add the cheese and serve.

SPROUTS

Seeds and grains are latent powerhouses of nutritional goodness and life energy. Add water to germinate them, let them grow for a few days in your kitchen and you will harvest delicious, inexpensive fresh foods of quite phenomenal health-enhancing value. The vitamin content of seeds increases dramatically when they germinate. The vitamin C can multiply five times within three days of germination – a mere tablespoon of soya bean sprouts contains half the recommended daily adult requirements of this vitamin. The vitamin B2 in an oat grain rises by 1,300 per cent almost as soon as the seed sprouts and by the time tiny leaves have formed it has risen by 2,000 per cent. Many sprouted seeds and grains also appear to have anti-cancer properties which is why they form an important part of the gentle natural methods of treating the disease.

When you sprout a seed, enzymes which have been dormant in it spring into action breaking down stored starch into simple natural sugars, splitting long-chain proteins into amino acids and converting saturated fats into free fatty acids. What this means is that the process of sprouting turns these seeds into foods which are very easily assimilated by your body when you eat them. Sprouts are, in effect, pre-digested and as such have many times the nutritional efficiency of the seeds from which they have grown. They also provide more nutrients ounce for ounce than any natural food known.

Another attractive thing about sprouts is their price. The basic seeds and grains are cheap and readily available in supermarkets and health-food stores – chickpeas, brown lentils, mung beans, wheat grains and so forth. And since you sprout them yourself with nothing but clean water, they become an easily accessible source of organically grown fresh vegetables, even for city dwellers. In an age when most vegetables and fruits are grown on artificially fertilized soils and treated with hormones, DDT, fungicides, insecticides, preservatives and all manner or other chemicals, home-grown-in-a-jar sprouts emerge as a pristine blessing – fresh, unpolluted and ready to eat in a minute by popping them into salads or sandwiches. As such they can be a wonderful health boon to any family concerned about the rising cost of food and the falling nutritional value in the average diet. Sprouts are the cheapest form of natural food around. Different sprouts mixed together will indeed support life all on their own. One researcher calculated that by eating sprouts alone you could live on less than 20p per person a day. While we would certainly never suggest that anybody live on sprouts alone, we think they are an ideal addition to the table of every family – particularly if the budget is tight.

By the way, children love them since they can help grow them themselves. And because they grow so quickly – the average sprout is ready for the table in about three days – it satisfies their impatience. The youngest member of our family, when he was two, used to carry a little bag of sprouts around with him, munching them between meals as some children do sweets.

D-I-Y Sprouting

When you discover how economical and easy it is to grow sprouts, you will want to have some on the go all the time. Once germinated you can keep sprouts in polythene bags in the fridge for up to a week – just long enough to get a new batch ready for eating. Most people grow sprouts in glass jars covered with nylon mesh held in place with an elastic band around the neck, but we have discovered an even simpler method which allows you to grow many more and avoids the jar method problem of seeds rotting due to insufficient drainage.

You will need the following:

seeds (e.g. mung beans)
seed trays with drainage holes. These are available from gardening shops and nurseries. (You can buy different sizes depending on the amount of sprouts you want to grow.)
a jar or bowl to soak seeds in overnight
a plant atomiser – available from gardening or hardware shops
a sieve
nylon mesh – available from gardening shops

1. Place two handfuls of seeds or beans in the bottom of a jar or bowl and cover with plenty of water. Leave to soak overnight.

2. Pour the seeds into a sieve and rinse well with water. Be sure to remove any dead or broken seeds or pieces of debris.

3. Line a seedling tray with nylon mesh (this helps the seeds drain better), and pour in the soaked seeds.

4. Place in a warm dark spot for fast growth.

5. Spray the seeds twice a day with fresh water in an atomiser and stir them gently with your hand in order to separate them.

6. After about three days place the seeds in sunlight for several hours to develop the chlorophyll (green) in them.

7. Then rinse in a sieve, drain well and put in a polythene bag in the fridge to use in salads, wok-frys etc.

There are many different seeds you can sprout – each with its own particular flavour and texture. Use the chart below as a guide to the variety of sprouts you can try.

Sprouting Chart

SMALL SEEDS soak 6–8 hours	Dry amount to yield 1³/4 pints (1 litre)	Ready to eat in	Length of shoot (approx.)	Growing tips and notes
Alfalfa	3–4 tbsp	5–6 days	1¹/2 in (3.5 cm)	Rich in organic vitamins and minerals, the roots of the mature plant penetrate the earth to a depth of 30–100ft (10–30m).
Fenugreek	¹/2C	3–4 days	¹/2 in (1 cm)	Have quite a strong 'curry' taste. Best mixed with other sprouts. Good for ridding the body of toxins.

| **Mustard**
no soaking
needed | 1/4C | 4–5 days | 1 in
(2.5 cm) | Can be grown on damp paper towels for at least a week; the green tops are then cut off with scissors and used in salads. |

LARGER SEEDS soak 10–15 hours	To yield 3 1/2 pints (2 litres)	Ready to eat in	Length of shoot (approx.)	Growing tips and notes
Adzuki beans	1 1/2C	3–5 days	1–1 1/2 in (2.5–3.5 cm)	Have a nutty 'legume' flavour. Especially good for the kidneys.
Chickpeas	2C	3–4 days	1 in (2.5 cm)	May need to soak for about 18 hours to swell to their full size. The water should be renewed twice during this time.
Lentils	1C	3–5 days	1/4–1 in (0.5–2.5 cm)	Try all different kinds of lentils – red, Chinese, green, brown. They are good eaten young or up to about 6 days old.
Mung beans	1C	3–5 days	1/2–2 1/2 in (1–5 cm)	Soak at least 15 hours. Keep in the dark for a sweet sprout. Put a weight (plastic bag filled with water and tied) on the beans to get long straight sprouts.
Soya beans	1C	3–5 days	1 1/2 in (3.5 cm)	Need to soak for up to 24 hours with frequent changes of water to prevent fermentation. Remove any damaged beans which fail to germinate.
Sunflower	4C	1–2 days	Same length as seed	Can be grown for their greens. When using sunflower seeds soak them and sprout for just a day. They bruise easily so handle with care.

GRAINS soak 12–15 hours	To yield 1³/4 pints (1 litre)	Ready to eat in	Length of shoot (approx.)	Growing tips and notes
Wheat	2C	2–3 days	Same length as grain	An excellent source of the B vitamins. The soak water can be drunk straight, or added to soups and vegetable juices.
Rye	2C	2–3 days	ditto	Has a delicious distinctive flavour. Good for the glandular system.
Barley	2C	2–3 days	ditto	As with most sprouts, barley becomes quite sweet when germinated. Particularly good for people who are weak or underweight.
Oats Soak 5–8 hours only	2C	3–4 days	ditto	You need whole oats or 'oat groats'. Oats lose much of their mucus-forming activity when sprouted.

Raw Power for Slimming

So useful is a Raw Energy way of eating for slimmers that the vast majority of people find when they begin eating this way they shed any excess weight slowly and naturally without ever having to count calories or restrict the quantities of energy rich foods such as seeds, grains and oils.

To anybody who has conscientiously fought (and frequently lost) the battle of the bulge, this can seem almost a miracle. It is not. It is simply a physiological result of the kind of re-balancing which takes place in the body on a high-raw diet. In our experience about 80 per cent of Raw Energy slimmers fall into this category. The other 20 per cent (to which, incidentally one of us belongs – Leslie) are only slightly less fortunate. For us to lose weight we have simply to cut back on the fattier foods such as the seed and nut cheeses and to avoid the richest of the salad dressings while eating as much as we like of the rest.

Slimming Secrets

Using the Raw Energy way of slimming works in several ways. First, it supplies your body with the highest complement of nutritional support it can get anywhere in the form of vitamins, minerals, easily assimilated proteins, and essential fatty acids so that you don't suffer the fatigue often linked with a calorie-restricted diet; neither do you end up with those dangerous sub-clinical vitamin deficiencies associated with off-again-on-again crash regimes. Second, the natural fresh foods we use in our recipes are rich in fibre. This is particularly important to slimmers since a high-fibre way of eating not only makes you feel full and satisfied – provided you are eating the right kind of soluble fibre (bran is *not* this kind, incidentally) – but it will also help your body stabilize blood-sugar levels and thereby reduce feelings of hunger. Some kinds of fibre such as pectin, which is found in good quantities in apples and some other fruits, help detoxify your body of poisonous wastes such as heavy metals like lead and aluminium.

Raw Energy eating centred around large quantities of fresh raw vegetables also offers enormous help to slimmers, thanks to the high potassium content of these foods and to their ability to make the body more alkaline. The by-products of the average Western diet rich in meat, sugar, coffee and processed foods, are highly acidic. Like stress, they tend to make the blood more acid. Taken over a long period of time such foods can put considerable strain on your body's natural mechanisms for maintaining its proper acid/alkaline balance.

Slimming itself tends to render your blood more acidic because the by-products of fat burners also tend to be acid. This can make slimmers feel nervous and irritable. The high potassium content of fresh raw vegetables and some fruits, and the ability these foods have to alkalinize the body, helps eliminate that unpleasant feeling of strain and nervousness slimmers know so well, and leaves you feeling well and calm as the pounds melt away.

An End to Cravings

Raw Energy slimming also works for many for whom no other slimming method has been successful, because it helps wipe out the cravings for foods that seem impossible to resist and which defeat many slimmers. You know the kind of thing: you go to the cupboard and reach for a biscuit to go with your tea and find yourself eating the whole packet. This results in feeling desperately guilty, in the sense that you feel hopeless, with 'no will power'. It also results in your trying to cut back on what you eat during the rest of the day to make up for all those extra calories. For many would-be slimmers this leads eventually to nutritional deficiencies and chronic fatigue which only make matters worse.

Such cravings – and the kind of uncontrollable eating which they spur – are often the result of a food intolerance, sometimes called a food allergy. As experts in food allergies will tell you – for complex biochemical reasons – you will tend to crave those foods to which you are intolerant or allergic, so that they become a kind of addiction. You simply can't stop eating them once you take a bite or two. This is a common problem – particularly among those who have experienced the off-again-on-again slimming.

The most frequently occurring intolerances centres on milk and milk products and wheat. They are foods which we therefore tend to eliminate from the menus of those people who are intent upon losing weight, but are not as fortunate as the 80 per cent who lose it naturally on a 75 per cent raw diet. They need extra help, and eliminating milk and wheat products brings this help to many. You will find the recipes in this section therefore contain no milk, cheese or yoghurt products, and no wheat flour of anything containing it. If you are one of the would-be slimmers who knows this craving pattern only too well you are likely to find that steering clear of these things will make all the difference in the world.

The Principles of Slimming
Simple. Here they are:
- Eat three meals a day.
- Make sure at least 50-75 per cent of what you eat is raw.

- Stress the energy-light-but-fibre-rich foods in your diet – particularly fresh raw vegetables, grains and pulses.
- Drink only *between* meals but then as much as you like.
- Chew your foods long and carefully.
- Indulge yourself in the splendour of many different dishes chosen not only from this section but others as well (leaving out milk and wheat products if you are not losing weight fast enough to please you).
- Enjoy your foods. Delight in them. Enjoy too the 'automatic will power' that seems to come when your body slowly re-balances itself through Raw Energy eating.

The Slimmer's Day

A sample menu would be as below:

SLIMMER'S PORRIDGE
PACKED LUNCH – CRUDITÉS, SPROUTS, DIP AND FRESH FRUIT
SLIMMER'S DINNER – PORTUGUESE PRAWNS with HOT SPICY SAUCE, BROWN RICE, GREEN SALAD AND FRESH FRUIT

The slimmer's choice of recipes in this book is almost as broad as any other's. Except for the rich dressings, cheeses and desserts which contain a lot of nuts and oils, the Raw Energy recipes are naturally ideal for slimming. The number of crunchy raw vegetables you can fill up on is unlimited. Be sure you dress them with one of our lighter dip-dressings such as Tofu, Raw Hummus or Curried Avocado and you'll be on the way to a slimmer you in no time.

Breakfast is very much like the Raw Energy muesli except that it includes the three seeds. These supply the essential fatty acids which everyone – even slimmers – need. Too many would-be skinnies avoid 'fat' in every form and end up with peeling skin and dull hair, as well as more serious deficiency problems. By including the right amount of good fats in your diet you will help avoid that feeling of your body 'needing' something while steadily shedding excess pounds. The oats and fruit in the porridge are an excellent source of fibre. You will find that the breakfast leaves you full and satisfied so that you are less troubled by hunger pangs and more able to stick to your regime.

Lunch is a packed lunch which includes lots of crudités, some sprouted beans, a tofu dip and a piece of fruit. For most people, especially those who go to work or school, lunch is the worst time of all for snacking on fattening foods. If you simply pack a box chock-a-block with good munchy foods you can reach for them at lunchtime (or snacktime) to satisfy your pangs.

Dinner is based around a large salad with a bowl of rice (or any other grain such as millet or buckwheat) and a little meat, fish, game or pulses etc. plus a little fresh fruit for dessert. The meal can consist of Green Salad with Spicy Tomato dressing which doubles up as a cocktail sauce for the Portuguese Prawns, a bowl of brown rice topped with chopped spring onions, and a bowl of black grapes.

BREAKFAST

Slimmer's Porridge

2 tbsp oatflakes (soaked overnight in water), 1 pear or apple (grated), 1 finely chopped banana, juice of 2 oranges, 1 tbsp minced three-seed mix (pumpkin, sunflower, sesame), pinch of cinnamon.

Combine the soaked oats with the fruit and orange juice and mix well. Sprinkle with minced 3 seeds and dust with the cinnamon. Enjoy!

As a variation try replacing the banana with other fruit such as a peach or a handful of strawberries. Or blend in a food processor to make a smooth porridge.

LUNCH

Fill a lunch box with the following:

Crudités

These vegetables and fruits make ideal crudités: carrot sticks, celery sticks, broccoli and cauliflower florets, rings or strips of red, yellow and green peppers, mangetout, diagonal slices of cucumber, courgette, thin slices of Jerusalem artichoke, white radish and kohlrabi, whole radishes, button mushrooms, spring onions, celery hearts, tomatoes, red and white cabbage slivers, apple wedges, orange segments, watercress, pineapple, olives.

A container of Tofu Dip (see page 358).

A small plastic container of mixed sprouts – e.g. mung, lentil and chickpea.

An apple or other piece of fruit.

DINNER

Prepare a Green Salad.
Arrange several cooked prawns over the salad.
Prepare the following sauce:

Spicy Hot Sauce/Dressing

This makes enough to use several times – store in a screw-top jar in the fridge.

6 ripe tomatoes, handful of basil leaves, 1 tsp Meaux mustard, 1 egg yolk, 2 tsp vegetable bouillon powder, few drops Tabasco, juice of ½ lemon, 1 tsp honey, 1 tbsp tomato puré, 1 tbsp minced onions, 1 crushed clove garlic

Process the tomatoes very finely. Add the other ingredients and blend well.

Bowl of hot brown rice
Bowl of black grapes
A glass of spring water with a twist of lemon if desired.

This is just one example of a slimming 75 per cent raw way of eating. There are plenty of other recipes – for salads, soups, dressings and desserts which a slimmer can feast on without feeling guilty or putting on weight.

Tea 'n' Treats

The worst health offenders in most ways of eating – particularly children's diets – are processed sweets made from refined sugar. Not only are they bad for teeth, they can cause more serious problems in children such as sub-clinical deficiencies or hyperactivity, and in adults can contribute to the development of degenerative diseases such as diabetes, arthritis and coronary heart disease. However, trying to get children to give them up is like pulling teeth from a hippopotamus. Far better to given them a wholesome alternative to replace those chocolate bars, biscuits and cakes.

In this section you will find recipes for all sorts of sweet treats, each made from nutritious ingredients – nuts, seeds, dried fruit, coconut, carob and honey – which can be served at tea time with one of our delicious shakes or smoothies, or taken to school in a lunch box to snack on. They are as tasty as they are wholesome.

Sweet Treats

The attractive little sweets can be wrapped in coloured paper and given in boxes as gifts for Easter, Christmas etc.

1C mixture of almonds and hazelnuts, 1C mixed dried fruit (such as date and apricot, peach and raisin, or sultana and pear), 1 tbsp honey, juice of 1 orange or ½C apple juice, dash of orange liqueur (optional), coconut flakes and sesame seeds

Put the nuts and the dried fruit in the food processor and chop thoroughly. Add the honey and enough fruit juice to make the mixture bind, plus a dash of orange liqueur if desired. Remove from the processor and roll into spheres the size of large marbles. Sprinkle a plate with the coconut flakes (toasted if desired) and sesame seeds and roll the balls in either one or both. Chill in the fridge and serve on a platter decorated with fresh fruit.

Carob and Apple Cake

This is wonderful Raw Energy cuisine replacement for Black Forest Gâteau!

1C sunflower seeds (or a 2:1 mixture of sunflower and sesame seeds), 1C carob powder, ½C dried coconut, ½C dried pitted dates, 3 apples, ½ tsp vanilla essence, 1 tsp allspice, apple slices or strawberries to garnish

Grind the seeds very finely. Add the carob powder, coconut and dates. Quarter and core the apples, then homogenize in the food processor with the dry ingredients. Add the vanilla essence and allspice. Spoon the mixture into a flat dish and leave to chill for a couple of hours in the fridge. Decorate with apple and/or strawberry slices before serving.

Shortcake Biscuits

These are great served as wafers with fresh fruit salad.

1C oatflakes, ½C dried dates, ⅓C dried coconut, 1–2 tsp vanilla essence, 1 tbsp honey

Process all the ingredients together well. Remove the mixture and squeeze off a small portion in your fist to make an oval shape. Press this flat on to a board, then turn it with a fish slice and flatten it on the other side. Place the wafers on a plate and chill in the fridge for at least half an hour.

Rocky Road Bananas

This is a great recipe if you have too many ripe bananas on your hands. Once frozen the bananas will keep for weeks – unless they are eaten immediately as in our house!

4 ripe bananas, ½–1C coarsely ground Brazil nuts, honey

Simply peel the bananas and skewer on to kebab or ice lolly sticks. Roll in honey and then in chopped nuts. Put on a freezer-proof plate and freeze until hard. Eat straight from the stick. If you prefer you can first slice the bananas crosswise, coat in honey and sprinkle with nuts, then freeze to make bite-sized treats.

As a variation try mixing a few tablespoons of carob powder into the honey to make chocolate coated bananas and then roll them in coconut, dates or nuts . . . or all three!

Porcupine Pineapple Chunks

A lovely idea for children's parties.

Cut a fresh pineapple into cubes and skewer on to cocktail sticks. Roll in clear honey and then coat with wheatgerm, sesame seeds or coconut. Chill and serve.

Yoghurt Lollies

The best ice-lollies are home-made. You can buy ice-lolly moulds and sticks in most department stores. We mix a large bowl or plain yoghurt with some frozen concentrated orange juice, then pour the mixture into the lolly moulds and freeze. You can also add fresh fruit and honey to natural yoghurt and blend it together to use, or simply freeze fresh fruit juices such as orange, grape, apple and pineapple.

Sorbets

The easiest way to make sorbets is with a sorbetière – a special machine which stirs the sorbet or ice cream as it freezes it. We have survived for many years without one by improvising . . .

Orange Sorbet Juice 8 oranges and then combine in the processor with 2 juicy seedless oranges which have been peeled and quartered. Add enough honey to sweeten and some nutmeg or ginger if desired. We sometimes like to add a grated peach or two to give the sorbet texture. Pour the mixture into ice-cube trays or a plastic lunchbox type container and freeze. Remove from the freezer and leave for about ten minutes to thaw slightly. Blend the mixture again immediately before serving and spoon into glass dishes or into empty halved orange shells.

Strawberry or Blackberry Sorbet Combine 3C berries with 2 bananas and a little honey. Follow the method as above. The bananas give a creamy texture to the sorbet.

Carob and Honey Ice Cream

This recipe is one of our family favourites. The combination of carob and honey we find unbeatable.

2 pints (about a litre) milk (we use goat's but you can use cow's or even skimmed milk if you like), 2 egg yolks, 3 tbsp granular lecithin (optional but very nice since it gives a creamier texture), 1C unheated carob powder, ½C clear honey, 1 tsp pure vanilla essence

Freeze the milk in a low flat plastic container. When frozen, remove from the freezer and let sit for about half an hour until it is just soft enough to slice into pieces. Put the egg yolks into the food processor, add about a cup of the frozen milk, the lecithin, carob powder, honey and vanilla, and blend thoroughly using the blade attachment.

Add the rest of the frozen milk and continue to blend until it is just mixed. (Don't overblend or you will make the ice cream too liquid.) Should it become too liquid simply return to the freezer for a few minutes then stir before serving. Serve immediately.

DRINKS

Cherry Whip (for 1)

1C natural yoghurt, ½C pitted black cherries, 2 tsp honey, double cream (optional)

Blend the yoghurt, cherries and honey and pour into a tall glass. Top with a spoonful of double cream and garnish with a pair of cherries hung over the edge of the glass. As a variation use strawberries or raspberries instead of cherries.

Banana Shake (for 1)

Peel and freeze a ripe banana, then chop it into fairly small pieces and blend with a cup of milk and a dash of vanilla essence. Sweeten with honey is desired.

Mocca Milk (for 1)

1C milk, ⅓C carob powder, 1 tsp instant cereal 'coffee' (chicory or ground barley based), 1 tbsp honey, vanilla essence, whipped cream and chopped pecans to top

Mix a little of the milk and the carob into a paste and put it in the blender with the rest of the milk, and 'coffee', the vanilla essence and the honey. Blend well and pour into a glass. Top with a little whipped cream and chopped pecans if desired.

Golden Smoothie (for 2)

2 oranges, 2 peaches, 1 banana, 1 tsp orange bitters or 1 tsp vanilla essence, 1tsp nutmeg, a little honey if desired

Peel the oranges and remove the pips. Homogenize in the food processor with the peaches and banana. Add the orange bitters or vanilla, the honey and the nutmeg. Combine well. Pour into two tall glasses with crushed ice and serve.

Garden Punch (for 4)

This is our favourite summer drink. To make a large jugful, you will need:

A large handful of fresh mint and lemon balm, 2C water, a handful of raspberries or blackcurrants, 1 orange, 1 lemon, 2C apples or grape juice, 1C pineapple or orange juice, 1C fresh elderflowers (de-stalked), honey, ice

Blend the fresh mint and lemon balm with the water and berries until the leaves are finely chopped. Add the grated rinds of the orange and lemon and leave the mixture to soak in the blender for at least fifteen minutes (preferably longer). Pour the other juices (apple or grape and pineapple or orange) into a jug. Squeeze the lemon and slice the orange. Add to the jug, then add the elderflower heads (these can be strained off later, but a few poured into the glasses with the drink are particularly attractive). Strain the mixture into the jug and discard the leaves, berry pulp and rinds. Sweeten with a little honey and chill. Serve in tall glasses with ice and fresh mint. You can also add a few other flowers from the garden such as orange blossom or lilac.

HERB TEAS

Our rich and delicious shakes and drinks are not for everybody. Kids love them but adults often prefer a simple tisane or herb tea which is light and refreshing, and can be drunk either hot with a little honey for sweetening, or made double strength, chilled and served in a tall iced glass. Herb teas make seductive and healthy alternatives to tea and coffee.

They come in two varieties – those which you take for medicinal purposes such as red sage as a gargle for a sore throat, dandelion to eliminate excess water from the body, lemon grass for indigestion and St John's Wort for skin problems – and those which you drink for pure pleasure. Some such as camomile and vervain (which are natural sedatives) and peppermint (which calms the digestive system) belong in both. Our favourites include lemon grass, lemon verbena, orange blossom, hibiscus and lime blossom.

You can either make your own from dried herbs or you can buy herb teas ready packaged in bags which you can use as you would ordinary tea bags – allowing them a little longer to steep. There are some wonderful herbal combinations on the market in these little bags – cinnamon and rose flavour, for instance, or apple and cinnamon. Or you can drink each tea separately.

Home-made Herb Teas

It takes about a tablespoon of the dried herbs (either a single herb or a mixture) to make two cups. Pour boiling water over it and let it steep in a pot for five to ten minutes, stirring every now and then to extract the full aroma. Now strain and serve with a slice of lemon and/or a little honey for sweetening. Sometimes we add cinnamon to herb teas and even a teaspoon of fresh cream.

In the summer drink them iced. We keep a teapot full of our favourite tea in the fridge drinking it often instead of eating snacks. But make it double strength and make sure if you want sweetening that you dissolve the honey in your tea before you chill it. Serve it with a twist of lemon in a tall glass with a sprig of mint or a pair of cherries sitting on the edge. Sometimes we even freeze small flowers such as honeysuckle, lilac or elderflower into cubes of ice and float these in the tea. Herbal flowers such as hibiscus give a beautiful red colour to chilled tea served in a tall glass.

RAW JUICES

Fresh pressed apple, grape or carrot juice is like nectar from the gods compared to the bottled variety you can buy. And raw juices have remarkable healing properties. They form the base of what we think is the best contribution the Germans ever made to renewing vitality and good looks. It's called the Rohsäfte-Kur. Europeans use it to revitalize themselves after a long winter when people eat too much, exercise too little and spend far too many hours in heated offices and houses. We use it when we are feeling 'dead' from too much stress, too little sleep or just simple fatigue. The Rohsäfte-Kur is simply a raw juice regime which you carry out over a day or even a few days to spring-clean your system and make you feel super-alive – mentally clear and beautifully receptive to things around you. It makes your skin glow and also quickly trims away a few excess pounds.

Raw juices are exceptionally rich in health-producing enzymes as well as vitamins, minerals and trace elements useful in restoring biochemical balance to the body. According to authorities on the Rohsäfte-Kur, raw vegetable and fruit juices accelerate the burning up and elimination of accumulated wastes. This is why a day or two on juices is the cornerstone of rejuvenation treatment at many expensive European health resorts.

Raw juices cannot be made in a food processor or blender. They require a special juice extractor – usually a centrifuge affair into which you feed the fruits and vegetables as it chops them and spins out their precious juices. Then you are left with the juice which you drink and the pulp which you toss into the compost. The health-promoting properties of fresh juices depends on their being drunk live – that is within a few minutes of being made – so that the oxidation process which sets in almost immediately does not destroy essential vitamins and enzymes. We find, however, that if you make a thermos full of juice and chill it immediately by filling it with ice cubes it will keep for several hours so you can take it to work or drink it throughout the day when you feel thirsty.

But raw juices are by no means only valuable because of their therapeutic properties. Some – such as fresh apple, grape and pineapple – are also the best tasting drinks we've ever come across. We often use raw juices to make delicious chilled soups as well, and, mixed together with mineral water, herbs and flowers, to make dazzling summer drinks.

If you are the fortunate owner of a juice extractor you should take the time to experiment a little to see which juices you prefer and what works best for you. We often make a base of carrot and apple – about half and half – to which we add smaller quantities of other juices such as cabbage, beetroot, berry, etc. Here are a few of the most common juices and some of their uses:

CARROT An excellent juice for alkalinising the system and therefore for countering stress. It is rich in carotene which the body turns into vitamin A – an important nutrient in protecting you from infection and early ageing. It also contains vitamins C, D, E and K. Useful for rebuilding healthy tissue and for treating skin problems.

APPLE Also a great cleanser, apple juice is believed to purify the blood and is useful as a general tonic. It contains vitamin C, many of the B complex vitamins, and lots of potassium and folic acid. Apple juice also helps overcome any sort of digestive upset.

CUCUMBER This juice is a natural diuretic – it encourages your body to get rid of excess water stored in the tissues. Drunk regularly it can be an aid to healthy hair and nails, thanks to its high sulphur and silicon content. We prefer cucumber juice mixed with, say, apple or carrot or both, since its taste is slightly insipid.

CABBAGE Not a nice tasting juice – cabbage needs to be mixed with carrot or something else as well – but it is also an effective internal cleanser and has been used medically as a treatment for healing stomach ulcers. Not useful for anyone with a sluggish thyroid, however, since cabbage can suppress thyroid activity somewhat.

GRAPE This juice is famous not only for its deliciousness but also for its natural sugars which are traditionally considered ideal for a short spring-clean regime. Warning: once you have tasted real fresh grape juice you will never again be content with the bottled variety!

Fabulous Feasts

The *Shorter Oxford English Dictionary* defines feast as 'A sumptuous meal or entertainment for many guests . . . something delicious to feed on.' We might add – a spread of food which not only tastes splendid, but is also seductive to the eye – a real hedonist's paradise. That is how we feel about what we call our Fabulous Feasts.

We delight in preparing numerous delicious Raw Energy dishes for our large family and many friends. We love to try out bounteous combinations of different tastes, colours and textures with the least possible excuse for celebration. It's challenging, it's fun, and it is always different. In this chapter we hope to give you some hint of just how splendid Raw Energy cuisine can be for parties and celebrations and to give you some of our favourite recipes for hors d'oeuvres, raw soups, main courses, side dishes and sweets. We hope you will like them as much as we do.

HORS D'OEUVRES

Mushroom Flower Cups

8–12 large button mushrooms, ¼C almonds (ground), 3 tbsp yoghurt, a squeeze of lemon juice, 1 tsp honey, 1 tsp dill seeds (roasted and ground), fresh parsley, vegetable bouillon powder, fresh mint

Remove the stalks of the mushrooms. Grind the almonds as finely as possible and mix with the yoghurt, lemon juice and honey. Add the ground dill seeds, a little chopped parsley and some bouillon powder. Spoon this mixture into the mushroom cups. Serve in twos and threes on little dishes garnished with mint sprigs.

Green Crêpes

These are stuffed lettuce leaves. The leaves need to be large and flexible so that they roll without splitting. For the stuffing we use finely chopped vegetables in a creamy egg or tahini mayonnaise (see page 375). A combination we particularly like is:

alfalfa sprouts, avocado, tomato, red pepper, spring onions, finely grated carrot or beetroot

Finely chop or grate the vegetables and mix them together with the dressing of your choice. Put spoonfuls of the mixture on to the lettuce leaves, roll them up and spear with a cocktail stick to hold in place.

Salad Kebabs

Skewered rows of different vegetable and fruit chunks make a very unusual and appetising starter. Make Salad Kebabs by skewering different things on wooden kebab sticks, such as:

button mushrooms, pitted olives, cherry tomatoes, pepper chunks, cucumber chunks, diced tofu or cheese, soaked dried prunes or apricots

Serve your skewers with a spicy dressing on a bed of shredded lettuce.

SOUPS
Carrot Chowder

This is one of our raw soups which can be warmed to just above blood heat (not over 40°C as this will kill the enzymes and some of the vitamins), or serve chilled.

¾C *walnuts/pecans, 8 carrots, juice of 3 oranges, 2C water, 1 egg yolk, 2 tsp vegetable bouillon powder, dash of white wine, ½ tsp fresh grated nutmeg, a few chopped chives to garnish*

Grind the nuts in a food processor. Add the carrots, roughly chopped, and re-process. Finally add the orange juice, water, egg yolk, bouillon, wine and nutmeg. Combine thoroughly. Serve at once or warm gently for a minute or two. Pour into individual bowls and top with chopped chives.

Gazpacho

This soup is particularly delicious served with 'croûtons' – roasted soya nuts or wheat and barley roasts (see page 372).

1 tbsp minced onion, 3 tomatoes, 1 red pepper, 2 small cucumbers, 3 egg yolks, 3 tbsp vinegar, 3 tbsp olive oil, 1 clove garlic, ½C tomato juice, 2 tsp vegetable bouillon powder, 1 tsp honey, dash of red wine (optional), 2 spring onions, fresh parsley and basil

Purée the onion, tomatoes, half the red pepper and one of the cucumbers in the blender or processor, then add the egg yolks, vinegar, olive oil, garlic, tomato juice, seasoning, honey and wine. Finely chop the spring onions, the other cucumber and the remaining red pepper and fresh herbs and add to the soup when you serve. Put the croûtons in a separate dish for people to help themselves.

Fresh Green Soup

2 avocados, 2C apple juice, 1–2C water (depending on how thick a soup you want), 2 lemons, 1 tsp vegetable bouillon powder, parsley, lovage, dash of white wine, the centre stalks of a head of celery

Peel and stone the avocados and process with the apple juice, water, 1 heaped teaspoon of chopped lemon rind, the juice of the lemons, bouillon, parsley, lovage and wine. Chop the celery stalks, including the leaves, and add to the soup. Blend well and serve garnished with a thin slice of lemon.

MAIN COURSES

The main course of our Fabulous Feasts is usually one of our Supersalads (see pages 362–86), perhaps with some rice, buckwheat, millet or a baked potato on the side. Sometimes we prepare a Sunburst Platter of crudités instead of a salad, and serve it with one of our vegetable loaves.

Sandstone Loaf

This dish has a beautiful pink/orange colour.

6 carrots, 2 stick celery, juice of ½ lemon, ¼C almonds, ¼C pumpkin seeds, 2 tbsp tahini, ½ onion, a handful of fresh parsley (or 1 tbsp dried), 2 tsp vegetable bouillon powders, 1 tbsp grated beetroot

Wash the carrots and celery. If the celery is stringy, peel away the tougher fibres with a knife. Roughly chop the carrots and celery and put into the food processor. Homogenize thoroughly, adding the lemon juice, and put into a separate bowl. Now grind the nuts and pumpkin seeds well. Add them to the carrot and celery mixture and stir in the tahini, finely chopped onion, parsley, bouillon and grated beetroot. Pack into a bread tin. Garnish with parsley leaves and almonds and serve from the tin.

Fermented Seed Loaf

This loaf is best fermented for several hours, so make it ahead of time.

½C almonds, ½C sesame seeds, 2 tbsp tamari, 1 clove garlic, basil, parsley, 1 tsp caraway seeds, ½–1C water, 1C chopped cauliflower or broccoli florets, 4 mushrooms, 2 sticks celery, radish slices to garnish

Finely grind the nuts and seeds. Add the seasonings – tamari, chopped garlic, basil, parsley, caraway seeds – and the water. Finely grate the cauliflower or broccoli and dice the celery and mushrooms. Mix all the ingredients together and pack into a bread tin. Cover with a tea towel and leave to ferment for several hours in a warm place. Add radish slices just before serving.

DESSERTS

Our desserts vary from the very simple, such as slices of fresh fruit sprinkled with ginger, to the more elaborate – our Stuffed Pineapple Salad or Raspberry Freeze Pie. Either way they are the crowning delight of a splendid feast and leave you feeling light and energized rather than bloated and drowsy.

Stuffed Pineapple

1 large pineapple, 1 orange, 1 mango or papaya (chopped), 1C raspberries or strawberries, 2 figs (fresh, or dried ones, soaked), dried coconut to garnish (optional)

Slice the pineapple in half lengthwise and remove the flesh from each half, leaving a ½ inch (1 cm) shell. Dice the flesh and mix it with the sliced orange, mango (papaya) and raspberries (halved strawberries). Finely chop the figs and add. Mix all the ingredients together and spoon into the pineapple shells. Sprinkle with dried coconut and serve.

Raspberry Fruit Freeze Pie

There are many variations that can be made on this theme – using different berries and fruit to fill the raw pie base.

Pie Base
1C *pitted dried dates, ½C almonds, ½C oatflakes, 1 tsp honey, a little water.*

Grind the dates and almonds as finely as possible in a food processor. Add the oats, honey and a little water and blend again. You need to add the water slowly to get the right consistency. You want the mixture to bind but not be sticky. Remove the base from the processor in a ball and flatten it into a pie dish with your fingers. As a variation you can add a tablespoon or two of coconut.

Pie Filling
2 *bananas, 2C raspberries, sherry, honey to sweeten*

Peel the bananas and chop into pieces about an inch (2.5 cm) or so thick. Freeze in a polythene bag with the raspberries until firm. Remove from freezer and blend the fruits together with a dash of sherry and a little honey to sweeten if desired. Pour into the pie crust and serve immediately garnished with a few banana slices or raspberries.

Strawberries and Cashew Cream

One of our favourite ways of eating strawberries is to pick them and leave their stalks on, then wash them well and serve with a bowl of yoghurt or sour cream and another of honey or raw sugar. Those with a sensitivity to milk can still enjoy strawberries and cream by making the own non-dairy 'cream' from cashew nuts, and pouring it over a bowl of ripe fresh strawberries.

Cashew Cream

1C nuts, ½C water or orange juice, 1–2 tsp honey, nutmeg

Blend the nuts and liquid as finely as possible in the blender or processor. Add a little honey and nutmeg and use as a topping for any fruit.

Cooking Foods

We recommend a diet of about 50 to 75 per cent raw food, so what about the other 25 per cent? Well, first you'll notice how cooked ingredients tend to creep into our raw recipes and salads: toasted sesame seeds or almonds for salad sprinkles; toasted coconut for sweet coatings; or roasted spices, such as dill, in dressings. Toasting nuts, seeds and spices brings out the subtle flavours of their aromatic oils and affords a greater range of tastes. For the rest we never allow cooked foods to become the focus of a meal, but rather enjoy them as 'side dishes'. And when we do cook something we pay great attention to *how* in order to preserve as much of its nutritional value as possible.

For instance, we would never dream of boiling a vegetable. Too many vitamins are destroyed in the process and too many minerals lost in the water as it is discarded. Vegetables are good steamed when you cook them. You can buy a steamer or improvise one using a colander placed in a saucepan to which you add a small amount of water. Even better – both for flavour and nutrition – are stir-fried vegetables done instantly in a wok so they remain crisp in the minutest quantity of olive or soy oil – oil which is never heated to the smoking point.

If we cook game or fish we cook it as slowly as possible to ensure it retains its natural juices and flavours. If you are a meat eater there is a lot to be said for game and fish. Unlike the meat from our domestic animals – beef, lamb, pork, etc. – both game and fish are low-fat foods. And of the fats they do contain, most are unsaturated. Also, because these creatures are not intensively farmed they do not contain the worrying array of chemicals our domestic animals now do.

Most of the foods we serve cooked, however, are not the meats and fishes, but rather what we call the 'peasant foods': soups, grains, pulses and porridges, Scottish oatcakes and dark German rye breads. We love thick country soups to go with our fresh salads and seed cheeses, particularly in winter. Many of these soups are based on the pulses – peas, beans, lentils – or the grains such as millet, oats, barley or brown rice. These foods are wonderfully rich in fibre and offer low-calorie, low-fat, sustained energy. And peasant foods are not expensive either. Neither are potatoes – one of the most underrated of all the natural foods. We bake ours in their jackets and eat them whole filled with home-made dips sprinkled with chives. New potatoes we steam gently without peeling and serve with chopped fresh mint and a little butter.

Change Slowly

One of the most important things to remember when adding more fresh raw foods to your diet is that it is best done slowly, slowly. This is for two reasons. First, changing your diet dramatically in any direction can cause digestive upset simply because the human body tends to rebel against whatever it is not accustomed to. Second – and more important – changes made slowly are far more likely to last.

Begin by making one meal a day a huge salad. Then notice how much better you feel in a week or two. As you look better, feel better and begin to discover for yourself the high energy potential such a way of eating offers, you will find yourself automatically including more and more fresh foods in your menu. This way the process of change becomes a natural evolutionary one from which not only you will benefit. Others will, too, as they notice how much Raw Energy is doing for you and become curious to follow your example.

Meanwhile enjoy your steak if you want it, or your cream buns. Neither of us would ever restrain ourselves from eating a piece of chocolate cake if we felt we wanted it. It is just that when you have tried enough pieces of chocolate cake and you remember what it feels like to each such foods, you find after a while you don't want them any more. Fresh strawberries dredged in coconut seem more appealing.

Here are some of the cooked foods we often eat and some of our favourite family recipes. We hope you like them.

The Beautiful Grains

Brown rice, wheat, barley, oats, millet, bulgar wheat and buckwheat are wonderful staple foods – high in fibre, a good source of protein when eaten with vegetables, and very filling. They are exceptionally good for athletes, slimmers and people who want to have sustained energy. The basic rule for cooking grains is you need about ½ cup of dry whole grains to serve each person.

The first thing to do with your grain is to wash it in cool water, using a strainer, to gently loosen the dust and small bits of dirt. Check to see there are no little bits of rock left. When the water through the strainer rinses clean they are ready to cook.

There are two basic ways of cooking whole or cracked grains. The first uses cold water mixed with the grain. The second adds boiling water to the grain. We prefer the boiling water method.

Sauté the grain either in a heavy dry pan or with the smallest amount of olive oil possible to brown it a little. (This is not necessary with rice or barley, but the others benefit greatly from it.) Now add boiling water, a handful of herbs and some vegetable bouillon powder to the pot and cover immediately. Bring to the boil and continue to cook at a simmer on the hob or (we prefer this) pop it all into a moderate oven to finish. (Do not stir the grains as this breaks them up and makes them stick in clumps.)

Every grain needs a slight different length of cooking time. Here are some guidelines.

BROWN RICE
Use twice as much water as rice and cook for 45 minutes. Usually we cook rice by simply adding cold water to the grain, bringing to the boil and then simmering.

MILLET AND BUCKWHEAT GROATS
One part to two parts water for 20–25 minutes. Millet can be cooked by the cold water method.

BULGAR WHEAT
This is wheat which has been cracked, toasted and steamed before you buy it. Use one part bulgar wheat to one and a half parts water. Cook for 20 minutes.

BARLEY
Use twice as much water as grain and cook for 1½ hours.

How do you serve grains? There are so many delicious ways: on their own with some herbs tossed in; with a few vegetables such as onions and mushrooms; cold leftover grains mixed into salads; and in thick nourishing country soups.

The Humble Pulses

One cup of beans, lentils or peas measured dry makes about four average servings. Like the grains, these inexpensive foods are also rich in fibre and have good sustaining power. And they come in such wonderful varieties – black beans, limas, kidney, soya, lentils of all sorts and colours, adzuki beans and chickpeas. These too we mix with salads sometimes. We also use them as the base for delicious soups and we casserole dishes with them lavished with fresh herbs.

Here's how to cook the pulses. We usually soak our pulses for several hours – or overnight in a cool place – before cooking them. This softens them and cuts the cooking time considerably. It also helps break down some of the starches they contain and renders them more digestible. After soaking throw the soak water away, put them in a pot, add three times as much water as pulses, bring to a boil and simmer until done. These too can be cooked in the oven instead of on top of the hob. We prefer oven cooking because you don't have to be so accurate about the time you take them out and because they are less likely to stick to the pot. Beans and lentils love carrots, onions and celery which we often add as well as herbs and seasoning. (Our famous vegetable bouillon powder works its magic here as well.)

Here's a brief guide to timings:

RED LENTILS
Twenty minutes (don't need soaking either).

SPLIT PEAS AND OTHER LENTILS
One hour.

OTHERS (EXCEPT SOYA BEANS)
One and a half hours.

SOYA BEANS
Two and a half hours.

CHICKPEAS
One and a half hours.

SOUPS

Our winter soups are hearty and full-bodied. We make them from whatever vegetables we happen to have, adding some millet, lentils, peas, rice, barley or whatever is handy for thickening, lots of fresh herbs from the garden or a few dried herbs, and perhaps some bouillon powder for seasoning. Here are three examples.

Thick Vegetable Soup

This makes enough for a good four to six servings.

4 carrots, 2 turnips, 2 leeks, 1 head celery, 1 parsnip, 2C garden peas, 1C runner beans, plus any other vegetables you happen to have (or substitutions), 2 tbsp olive oil, 1 tbsp vegetable bouillon powder, 2 bay leaves, 3 pints (1.5 litres) stock or water, ³⁄₄C brown rice or millet, fresh parsley

Wash and peel the vegetables. Cut root vegetables into small cubes, the leeks first lengthwise four to six times then across so you get tiny pieces. Add oil to pot and sauté leeks. Then add chopped celery, carrots, and turnips, putting the lid on to allow them to sweat for five minutes. Now add the vegetable bouillon, bay leaves, stock or water (boiling) and the rice, and allow to cook for 30 minutes. Now add peas and beans and cook for another 15 minutes. Sprinkle with chopped parsley and serve.

Borscht

This serves four to six people well.

3 raw beetroot (with their tops if possible), 1 medium onion, 3 carrots, ½ small cabbage, 2 tbsp olive oil, 2 pints (about a litre) stock or water, 1 tbsp vegetable bouillon powder, juice of 1 lemon, 3 tbsp honey, 1 cup of thick yoghurt or sour cream, a dash of nutmeg

Wash vegetables – do not peel – and cut them into small strips. Retain half of one beetroot which you will add grated to the soup later. Heat oil in pot and sweat beet-root and onion for five minutes, then add the rest of the vegetables, including the sliced beet greens, and stew for another five to ten minutes, stirring occasionally. Add boiling stock or water – together with bouillon powder, and cook vegetables until tender. Now add lemon juice, grated beetroot and honey and cook for another five minutes, then serve topped with the thick yoghurt or sour cream and grated nutmeg.

Potato Soup

This, too, serves four to six people.

6 medium potatoes, 2½ pints (scant 1.5 litres) water or stock, 1 tsp vegetable bouillon powder, 1C sliced, chunked or diced vegetables (such as leeks, celery, carrot, swede, green beans, peas, etc.), herbs such as marjoram, winter savory, basil and garlic), garnishes (such as sliced spring onions, chopped hard-boiled egg, chives, water-cress, or grated hard cheese)

Scrub potatoes and wash vegetables, cutting them into medium-sized chunks. Cover the potatoes with the water or stock to which the bouillon has been added and boil until tender. Remove from heat and blend in a food processor until smooth. Now sauté the vegetables (cut into small pieces) and add them to the potato mixture along with the herbs, and cook for five minutes. Sprinkle with your garnishes and serve.

WOK FRYING

The most delicious way of all to cook vegetables is à la Chinoise – in a wok or frying pan. It is quick, simple and a lot of fun to do. Here's how.

Use no more than 2 tbsp soy or olive oil, then take whatever vegetables you happen to have. A good combination is:

a handful of cashews, cauliflower (broken into florets), mangetout (topped and tailed), onions (cut into rings), red pepper (diced), mushrooms (sliced), spring onions (spiked – their green part slit lengthwise), tamari

Put the oil into your pan and heat. Add cashews on their own and brown, then add vegetables which take longest to cook such as onions and cauliflower. Sauté for two to three minutes, turning constantly. Now add the rest of the vegetables and continue to toss them in the pan for another three to five minutes. Add a little tamari and serve.

A Guide to Raw Energy Shopping

Not only are the methods of food preparation and the equipment you need different in preparing Raw Energy foods, so is the shopping. You will find your larder stocked with a whole new set of ingredients – particularly if until now you have been living on the average Western fare of fast foods or meat and two veg. The delicious foods which you will use for most of these recipes are not only good for you, most of them are very tasty on their own – grains and legumes, nuts and seeds, fruits, vegetables and herbs.

These foods can either be bought at great cost, or, if you shop around, very cheaply. Because we have a large family we buy many of our fruits in crates from the wholesaler at less than half the price you pay in your greengrocer. You can pay dearly for nuts and seeds, grains and pulses in some health-food stores where they come in tiny packages (and are often not very fresh either). But pulses can be bought cheaply in the average supermarket and nuts, grains and dried fruit can be purchased at reasonable cost from many of the new whole-food emporiums which are appearing around the country. Obviously the more you buy at one time the cheaper they are. Be sure to refrigerate your nuts after purchase to keep their oils from going rancid. And if ever you buy a package of anything which you find on returning home is not absolutely fresh, take it back and complain. That is the only way to protect yourself while improving the quality of what is being sold.

Here is a brief guide to stocking a Raw Energy larder to give you some idea of just how much variety you have to choose from.

First of all the fresh fruits and vegetables which *must* be refrigerated.

Fruits

Fruits are often divided into different groups depending on which combine best together for digestion.

'ACID'
Orange, lemon, grapefruit, lime, strawberries, pineapple, pomegranate, plums (and prunes), blackberries, raspberries, black and red currants, tangerine, kumquats, ugli.

'SUB-ACID'
Apple, apricot, figs, grapes, mango, papaya, pear, peach, cherries, blueberries, nectarines, kiwi, lychees, passion fruit.

'SWEET'
Banana, dates, persimmon, most dried fruit.

'MELONS'
Watermelon, cantaloupe, honeydew, cassaba.

Fresh Vegetables

There are basically three categories: leaves, roots and fruit vegetables.

LEAVES
Lettuce (Cos, Chinese, iceberg, Webb's Wonder, lamb's or corn salad, romaine, red or radicchio, Boston), cabbage (red, white, green), cress (watercress, land cress, mustard and cress), spinach, endive (curled, round-leaved, French), chicory, beet tops, dandelion leaves, kale, Brussels sprouts, ruccola

ROOTS
Carrot, beet, radish (horseradish, white radish), turnip, parsnip, celeriac, Jerusalem artichoke, kohlrabi, salsify, fennel.

FRUIT VEGETABLES
Cauliflower, avocado, broccoli, onions (leeks, spring onions, red onions, shallots), celery, peppers (red, green, yellow), tomatoes, cucumbers (courgettes, aubergine,

young marrows, squash), peas and beans (legumes), mushrooms (fungus).

Cereals

These figure in many of our mueslis and savoury recipes. Those we use most often are: wheat, rye, oats, barley and millet. These can be bought in 'flake' or cut form and soaked to use in mueslis, or bought whole and sprouted for salads.

Millet is a particularly good grain and worth getting to know. It is the only alkaline grain and the only grain that contains all eight essential amino acids. It can be used sprouted, or cooked.

Buckwheat, often classified as a grain, is in fact a member of the Polygonacea family which includes rhubarb and sorrel. It is the triangular seeds of this plant that are sold. They are often pre-roasted, but can be bought raw. As with millet they can be eaten cooked or sprouted.

Oils

Buying good oil is very important. The best kind is fresh unrefined, cold-pressed extra virgin olive oil. This is because it is a monounsaturated oil and as such much more stable than the polyunsaturates from corn, peanuts, sunflowers or safflower seeds. It is also extracted from the fruit by mechanical pressing rather than by heat and chemical processing methods. As such the fatty acids it contains are in a form that your body can make good use of for building cell walls, making hormones and keeping nerve sheaths strong and healthy. In heat-processed oils, such as most you find on supermarket shelves, these usable 'cis' acids have been chemically changed into 'trans' fatty acids which can not only be actively harmful, they can actually block the uptake of any essential 'cis' fatty acids in the rest of your diet as well.

Olive oil is good and adds a distinctive flavour to salad dressings. It is quite heavy, though, and some people prefer a lighter oil. Soya oil and **walnut oil are lighter,** and both are delicious too. Walnut oil is wonderful (but it's expensive).

Nuts

When buying nuts make sure they are really fresh. The rancid oils in old nuts are harmful to the stomach, retard pancreatic enzymes, and destroy vitamins. If nuts are fresh and whole (unbroken) you can buy a kilo or so at a time and, provided they are kept airtight in a cool dry place (best in your refrigerator), they will keep for a few months. You can even freeze them. It is a good idea to buy a few different kinds. Then if you mix them you will get a good balance of essential amino acids. You will also have more variety in your recipes.

Choose from: almonds, Brazils, cashews, coconuts (fresh or desiccated), hazels, macadamia nuts, peanuts (strictly speaking a legume), pecans (similar to walnuts, but less bitter), pine kernels, pistachios, tiger nuts and walnuts.

Seeds

Again be sure you buy really fresh seeds with no signs of decay. The three seeds which provide such a valuable combination of protein and essential fatty acids are sunflower, pumpkin and sesame. Other seeds worth trying, mainly for seasoning, are poppy, celery, caraway, dill, fennel, and anise. The last four make good snacking 'sweets', separate or in combination. In the eighteenth and nineteenth centuries people used to carry a mixture of these seeds in their pockets whenever they went out to meetings and would munch on them to keep their appetites at bay.

Legumes and Other Sprouts

Remember, all whole seeds, grains and sprouts are living things and should be stored and handled with care.

Here are a few kinds of sprouts (for more ideas see page 384): alfalfa seeds, adzuki beans, mung beans, lentils, fenugreek, radish, chickpeas, soya beans and peas.

Special Foods

CAROB (ST JOHN'S BREAD) Carob powder/flour is a superb chocolate substitute – and good for you too. Unlike chocolate it does not contains caffeine. Instead it is full of minerals – calcium, phosphorus, iron, potassium, magnesium and silicon – as well as vitamins B1, B2, niacin and a little vitamin A plus some protein. Carob powder is often sold toasted, but the best kind is raw. It is lighter in colour than the cooked kind. It can be bought from most healthfood shops and used to make chocolate drinks, desserts and treats.

TOFU This is soya bean curd made from soya milk. All soya bean products are very high in protein and low in carbohydrates so they make a good food for dieters. Soya beans also contain a high amount of lecithin which fights the build-up of cholesterol deposits and is needed for the proper functioning of the brain and nervous system. Soya is a highly alkaline food. Both soya milk and tofu can be found in healthfood stores. They don't have a strong flavour, but taste slightly nutty and are quite palatable. One disadvantage of soya products is that, unless they are cooked or made from the sprouted beans, they contain phytic acid which binds the important mineral zinc and prevents its absorption.

WHEATGERM A delicious and valuable food high in vitamins E and B complex. Like molasses, it is the 'goodness' that is removed from the original product (in this case wheat) when it is refined. It should be bought raw, vacuum packed, not 'toasted', and then refrigerated to keep it fresh and can be used liberally sprinkled on salads, mueslis, desserts and so forth.

COCONUT Besides fresh coconut you can buy natural coconut in two forms – flaked or shredded. Make sure the kind you buy has not been sweetened with sugar or glucose syrup as so many are. For most uses we prefer the shredded. We sprinkle it on mueslis and use it a lot in treats. It keeps well for weeks in the refrigerator.

DRIED FRUIT When buying these be sure they are not dipped in glucose (figs and banana chips as well as pineapple, mango and papaya usually are). Also, try to find sun- rather than sulphur-dried fruit: raisins, sultanas, currants, apricots (look out for the unsulphured, unpitted Hunza ones), peaches, prunes, pears, figs, dates and bananas.

Sweeteners

HONEY This makes a wonderful substitute for sugar in drinks and desserts. There are so many sorts ranging from very mild – such as acacia or orange blossom – to very strong, such as Mexican honey or Tupolo from pines. If you don't like one kind, don't be put off, there are plenty of others to try. Clear honeys are best for drinks whereas set honeys, such as clover, are nice on breads. The best honeys are those labelled 'organic' as many commercial ones are made using sugar-fed bees. Honey contains many useful trace minerals.

MOLASSES This is one of the 'super-foods'. It is the left-over bulk from sugar refinement and is as good as bleached sugar is bad. It contains all the minerals and vitamins that are taken out of processed sugar. It is particularly rich in B complex vitamins and minerals. Much molasses is quite overpowering in its flavour and tends to have an unpleasant sulphur tang. This is because sulphur has been added in the sugar-extraction process. Unsulphured molasses, however, is quite delicious and can be eaten straight off the spoon. If kept in the refrigerator it becomes firm and thick and is wonderful on muesli or in yoghurt and spread on bread.

The best kind of sugar is raw cane or molasses sugar as it is unrefined. Billington's Golden Granulated sugar is the best. But with honey and molasses, you really don't need to use sugar and you're better off without it. Also, when you eliminate sweet foods from your diet you find that you really don't want them any more.

Herbs and Spices

Remember to buy spices in small quantities from shops with a good turnover, as they soon lose their freshness. The most flavourful herbs are freeze-dried, but these are hard to find. Vacuum-sealed herbs are a good bet. Remember to store your herbs and spices in the dark as the light affects their potency (so much for herb and spice racks!). For the sake of flavour it is best to buy whole spices and grind them yourself when needed in a coffee grinder or with a pestle and mortar. If you've never ground your own you'll be amazed at the splendid aroma and taste. With fresh herbs, wash and dry them well, then store in sealed polythene bags in the salad compartment of your fridge.

The list that follows contains many seasonings that you will find in the recipes.

'SWEET' SPICES (for fruit salads and dressings, desserts and ethnic dishes)
Allspice, angelica, aniseed, cardamom, cinnamon, cloves, coriander, ginger, nutmeg and mace.

'SAVOURY' SEASONINGS (for salads, soups and raw main dishes)
Basil, bay, caraway seeds, cayenne pepper, celery seeds, chervil, chilli powder, chives, coriander leaves (fresh), cumin, curry powder, dill, fennel, garlic, horseradish, juniper berries, kelp, lemon balm, lovage, marjoram, mint, mustard seeds, onion, oregano, paprika, parsley, pepper, poppy seeds, rosemary, sage, savory, sorrel, tarragon, thyme.

SAVOURY SEASONING POWDER This seasoning is useful for those times of panic when you just don't know what to add to give your dish the 'something' that it needs. Our rescue remedy that we wouldn't be without is a wonderful vegetable bouillon powder made by Marigold Health Foods Limited, Unit 10, St Pancras Commercial Centre, 63 Pratt Street, London NW1 0BY. Tel: 0171 267 7368, and called simply *Swiss Bouillon Powder*. Buy the low-salt variety. It has more flavour. We use it in dressings, sauces, ferments, soups, seed and nut dishes – just about everywhere.

Condiments and Other Flavourings

Some other useful additions for the larder shelf:

MUSTARD Mustard can be bought in dry or paste form. The dry powder is sometimes useful in dressings. We think the most delicious mustards are French. They are milder and more aromatic than English mustard. Moutarde de Meaux is particularly delicious and is great in dressings for all sorts of salads. Dijon and Bordeaux are also nice.

TAHINI (preferably unroasted). This is made simply from finely ground sesame seeds and has many uses including tahini mayonnaises, as an addition to many seed and nut dishes, and mixed with honey as a topping for fruit and desserts.

TAMARI This is a type of soya sauce made from fermented soya beans, but unlike soya sauce it contains no wheat. Unfortunately it does contain sea salt, so it should be used in moderation. Nevertheless, it is good for giving a 'Chinese' taste to dishes as well as a rich flavour to bland dressings or sauces.

YEAST EXTRACT This can be used as a substitute for 'vegetable bouillon'. It is rich in B complex vitamins, but very salty, so it should also be used in moderation.

VINEGAR Apple cider vinegar is the best as it contains malic acid which is helpful in the digestive process.

VANILLA ESSENCE Try to find real vanilla essence rather than the more common vanilla flavouring which is synthetic. Used in nut milks or yoghurt drinks and desserts, it gives a delicious warm flavour.

Raw Food Cautions

Some foods should not be eaten raw. Pulses and beans, for instance, have a number of negative attributes. Soya beans, broad beans and kidney beans contain a trypsin inhibitor. This substance blocks the action of certain enzymes in the body so that not all of the essential amino acids the beans contain can be used. Many years ago researchers discovered that soya beans would not support life unless they were cooked for several hours. In the human body the trypsin inhibitor is believed significantly to alter the nutritional value of proteins, rendering them virtually useless for us. When these foods are cooked or sprouted, however, the trypsin inhibitor is eliminated and they are rendered good to eat.

Chickpeas and green peas also contain a trypsin inhibitor but one which is not neutralized by heat, and peas contain a haemaglutin which resists heat. Haemaglutins inhibit growth in an animal by combining with the cells in the lining of the intestine and blocking nutrient absorption. But the trypsin inhibitor in chickpeas is rendered harmless when they are sprouted and the harmful elements in peas occur in such small quantities that many people eat them both raw and cooked without any adverse effects. Eating raw lima beans or red kidney beans, however, has been known to cause death.

The Brassicas

Cabbage, Chinese cabbage, watercress, kale, swede, turnip, rape, Brussels sprouts and mustard belong to a genus called Brassica. They contain compounds called thioglucosides which disrupt the functions of the thyroid gland and have been shown to contribute to the development of goitre. Similarly, drinking the milk of animals who have been grazing on these plants can interfere with thyroid function. But the negative effect of the Brassicas is eliminated provided you have adequate iodine in your diet. It is something we never worry about for it is only people deficient in iodine who suffer these effects.

The Raw Egg

People are often cautioned against eating raw eggs. Provided they are free-range and salmonella-tested, raw egg yolks are fine but the white of an egg contains avidin, a substance which combines with biotin and prevents it from reaching the blood. This could lead to a biotin deficiency. In a young man who ate many raw egg whites on their own symptoms such as scaly skin, anaemia, anorexia, nausea and muscle pains developed. The albumen in the egg white also dissolves in water and can easily enter the bloodstream undigested resulting in allergies. This is, of course, only in extreme cases and is far more likely if someone is eating the raw egg whites on their own rather than in combination with the yolks.

We generally prefer to use only the raw yolk in our recipes. However we do not think twice about preparing a delicious egg nog occasionally. It is simply a question of moderation.

Sprouting Improves Safety and Quality

Because of the massive enzyme release which occurs when a seed or grain is sprouted the nutritional quality of a sprout is extremely good as well as its 'safety'. These enzymes not only neutralize such factors as trypsin inhibitors but also destroy other substances which can be harmful such as phytic acid. Phytic acid, which occurs in considerable quantity in grains, particularly wheat, tends to bind minerals so that the digestive system cannot break them down for assimilation. When a grain is sprouted this mineral-binding capacity is virtually eliminated.

Did You Know That . . .

Athletes Can Improve Their Performances on Raw Foods
Professor Karl Eimer, director of the First Medical clinic at the University of Vienna, put top athletes into a high-intensity training programme for a fortnight and then suddenly changed their diet to one of entirely raw foods. His athletes grew stronger, faster and more supple.

Raw Foods are a Boon to Slimmers
The uncooked fibre which they contain decreases the amount of fat absorbed during digestion, creates a feeling of fullness and satisfaction, and spring-cleans the body of waste products that can make you feel tired. Raw foods also decrease food sensitivity reactions which lead many people to over-eat from cravings, raise energy levels and, thanks to their alkalinizing quality, enhance your ability to deal with stress.

The High-Raw Diet Benefits the Whole Person
It offers the perfect and complementary combination of all the nutrients essential for maximum vitality, both of the body as a whole and on a cellular level. Raw foods increase the micro-electrical potentials of cells, improving your body's use of oxygen so that both muscles and brain are energized.

Raw Foods are Perfect Spring-Cleaners of the Body
They help you eliminate stored wastes and toxins which interfere with the proper functioning of cells and organs and lower your energy levels.

Raw Foods are Central to the Gentle Approach to Treating Cancer

A typical anti-cancer regime, used effectively for almost 100 years in Europe, consists of organically grown foods and juices made from them. On this regime 80–90 per cent of foods are eaten raw.

Our Bodies React to Cooked Foods as an Invasion

Research done at the Institute of Clinical Chemistry in Lausanne showed that the body recognizes cooked and processed foods as invaders. They trigger the body's defence system – sending white blood cells into the intestine as soon as the food enters the mouth. Eating raw foods leaves your white blood cells free for other tasks and saves the body the effort of a defensive action, thereby strengthening its resistance to disease.

Diabetics and Arthritics Have Been Cured on Raw Food Diets

The tradition of treating degenerative diseases on a high-raw diet is a long one. At some of Europe's most famous clinics, such a diet is still used to lower blood pressure and cholesterol levels and treat many other major and minor problems.

Resources

Green Foods

Lifestream spirulina and other good green products are available mail order from Xynergy Products, Lower Elsted, Midhurst, West Sussex GU29 9JT. Tel: 01730 813642. Fax: 01730 815109.

Chlorella is available in capsule form from Solgar Vitamins Ltd, who also do an excellent powdered green supplement Green & More. For your local stockist contact: Solgar Vitamins Ltd, Solgar House, Chiltern Commerce Centre, Ashridge Road, Chesham, Buckinghamshire HP5 2PY. Tel: 01494 791691. Fax: 01494 792729.

Wheat-grass juice in powdered form is available from Malcolm Simmonds Herbal Supplies, 3 Burton Villas, Hove, East Sussex BN3 6FN. Tel: 01273 202401.

Green Magma, the dried juice of young barley leaves, is available from good healthfood stores.

Herbs An excellent supplier of tinctures, fluid extracts, loose dried herbs and the Schoenenberger plant juices is Phyto Pharmaceuticals Ltd, 3 Kings Mill Way, Hermitage Lane, Mansfield, Nottinghamshire NG18 5ER. Tel: 01623 644334. Fax: 01623 657232. Minimum order £10.

Another good source is Malcolm Simmonds Herbal Supplies, 3 Burton Villas, Hove, East Sussex BN3 6FN. Tel: 01273 202401.

Herbs are also available from Solgar Vitamins Ltd, Solgar House, Chiltern Commerce Centre, Ashridge Road, Chesham, Buckinghamshire HP5 2PY. Tel: 01494 791691. Fax: 01494 792729.

Honey The Garvin Honey Company have a good selection of set and clear honeys from all over the world. These can be ordered from The Garvin Honey Company Ltd, Garvin House, 158 Twickenham Road, Isleworth, Middlesex TW7 7LD. Tel: 020 8560 7171.

The New Zealand Natural Food Company have a fine range of honey, including organic honey, in particular Manuka honey, known for its anti-bacterial effects. The New Zealand Natural Food Company Ltd, Hold Close, Highgate Wood, London N10 3HW. Tel: 020 8444 5660.

Linseeds or Flaxseeds Linusit Gold are vacuum-packed and very good. Grind the seeds in a coffee grinder and sprinkle on cereals, salads, in yoghurt or in drinks. Or put dry into a blender, grind them and pour on your fresh juice. Available from healthfood stores.

Other good linseeds can be bought from Higher Nature Limited, The Nutrition Centre, Burwash Common, East Sussex TN19 7LX. Tel: 01435 882880.

Linseed oil can be obtained in capsules from Biocare, 17 Pershore Road, Birmingham B30 3EE. Tel: 0121 433 3727.

Marigold Swiss Vegetable Bouillon Powder This instant broth based on vegetables and sea salt is available from health food stores or direct from Marigold Foods, Unit 10, St Pancras Commercial Centre, 63 Pratt Street, London NW1 0BY. Tel: 020 7267 7368. It comes in regular, low-salt and vegan forms; the low salt and vegan are better as they have more flavour. The low-salt form is excellent for making spirulina broth.

Organic Foods The Soils Association publishes a regularly-updated National Directory of Farm Shops and Box Schemes which costs £3, including postage, from The Organic Food & Farming Centre, 86 Colston Street, Bristol BS1 5BB.

Organic Meat For excellent venison and wild boar in cuts of meat, burgers and sausages, low in fact and full of taste: Longwood Farm Organic Meats, Tudenham St Mary, Bury St Edmunds, Suffolk IP28 6TB. Tel: 01638 717120.

Sea Plants such as kelp, dulse, nori, kombu can be bought from Japanese grocers or macrobiotic health shops.

Soya Milk The best soya milk we have come across is called Bonsoy, and is available from good healthfood stores.

Water As you know getting pure water can be difficult. One in ten of us drink water which is contaminated with poisons above inernational standards. I have finally found a water purifier which I think is good – the Fresh Water FW 1000. It removes more than 90 per cent of heavy metals, pesticides, hydrocarbons such as benzyne, trihalmethanes, chlorine, oestrogen and bacteria, without removing essential minerals like calcium. It uses a six stage process to remove the wide variety of pollutants, unlike carbon based water filters, and it is housed in stainless steel. It can be cleaned if the flow rate slows down and comes with a 10 year guarantee plus after sales service. Their address is: Carlton

House, Aylmer Road, Leytonstone, London, E11 3AD. Tel: 020 7558 7495. Fax: 020 8556 9270. They are also recommended by ION and many leading allergy clinics.

Special Jucing Equipment

The Champion Masticating Juicer

Veteran juicers wax lyrical about the virtues of the Champion, an inde-structible, American juicer that some people claim makes better juice than any centrifugal extractor can because its masticating action is more effective at 'trituration', the process of splitting open the fibres of the plant matter and liberating its nutrients in the form of juice. The Champion is basically a rotating cutter on a shaft, which expels dry pulp from its snout at one end as the juice is drained through a nozzle underneath.

Expensive, the Champion is guaranteed for five years and can well last a lifetime, easily repaying the investment in the long run. Available from The Nutri Centre, 7 Park Crescent, London W1N 3HE. Tel: 020 7436 5122.

At the other end of the scale, Moulinex do an inexpensive centrifu-gal juicer which is good.

The Vita-Mix Total Nutrition Centre

A turbo-charged, super-efficient blender with indestructible stainless steel blades and an extremely powerful motor, the TNC is dynamite! It's the only machine that is properly able to make the fibre-rich juices – the kind of molecular or *total*, juicing – discussed in Book Two, Chapter Seven. It is also effective for making cereal grass juices (which should be strained before drinking to remove indigestible cellulose fibres). The TNC not only makes juice, but can also be used to make soups and ice cream. The Super TNC can even be used to mix whole-grain bread. These American machines are expensive, but owning one could change your life. Contact Vita-Mix in the USA for the name of a local distributor. Vita-Max Corporation, 8615 Usher Road, Cleveland, OH 44138, USA. Tel: 001 216 235 4840.

SPROUTING

All you need to start your own indoor germinating 'factory' are a few old jars, some pure water, fresh seeds/grains/pulses, and an area of your kitchen or a windowsill which is not absolutely freezing.

Home-made sprouters

There are two main ways to sprout seeds – in jars and in seed trays. Jars are traditional, but we find seed trays easiest and best.

A simple, and cheap sprouter can be anything from a bucket to a polythene bag. The traditional sprouter is a wide-mouthed glass jar. The easiest and least fussy way to use them is to use open jars and to cover a row of them with a tea towel to prevent dust and insects from getting in.

Start here

- Put the seed/grain/pulse of your choice, for example mung, in a large sieve. Remember that most sprouts give a volume about eight times that of the dry matter. Remove any small stones, broken seeds or loose husks and rinse your sprouts well.
- Put the seeds in a jar and cover with about 10cm of pure water. Rinsing can be done in tap water, but the initial soak, where the seeds absorb a lot of water to set their enzymes in action, is best done in filtered or boiled and then cooled spring water, as the chlorine in tap water can inhibit germination – and is also not very good for you.
- Leave your sprouts to soak overnight.
- Pour off the soak-water. If none remains then you still have thirsty beans on your hands, so give them more water to absorb. The soak-water is good for watering houseplants. Some people like to use it in soups or drink it straight, but we find it extremely bitter. Also, the soak-water from some beans and grains contains phytates – nature's insecticides, which protect the vulnerable seeds in the soil from invasion by micro-organisms. These phytates interfere with certain biological functions in man including the absorption of many minerals (for example zinc, magnesium and calcium), and are therefore best avoided. The soak-water from wheat, however, known as 'rejuvelac', makes a wonderful liquid for preparing fermented cheese and is very good for you.
- Rinse the seeds by tipping them into a large sieve and rinsing them well before replacing them in the jar. Be sure that they are well drained as too much water may cause them to rot. Repeat this process morning and night for most sprouts. During a very hot spell they may need a midday rinse too.
- Return the sprouter to a reasonably warm place. This can be under the sink, in an airing cupboard or just in a corner not too far from a radiator. Sprouts grow fastest and best *without* light and in a temperature of about 21°C (70°F).

- After about 3–5 days your sprouts will be ready for a dose of chlorophyll, depending on what kind you are growing. Alfalfa thrive on a little sunlight after they've grown for two or three days but mung beans, fenugreek and lentils are best off without it. Place the sprouts in the sunshine – a sunny windowsill is ideal – and watch them develop little green leaves. Be sure that they are kept moist and that they don't get too hot and roast!
- After a few hours in the sun most sprouts are ready to be eaten. Optimum vitamin content occurs 50–96 hours after germination begins. They should be rinsed and eaten straight away or stored in the refrigerator in an airtight container or sealed polythene bag. Some people dislike the taste of seed hulls such as those that come with mung sprouts. To remove them simply place the sprouts in a bowl and cover with water. Stir the sprouts gently. The seed hulls will float to the top and can be skimmed off with your hand.

Make it big

Now for our favourite and simplified method using seed trays. Leslie finds that, with the great demand of her family for living foods, the jar method simply doesn't produce enough. Also, tray sprouts need only a splash of water each day. This is an extremely simple way to grow even very large quantities easily.

Take a few small seed trays (the kind gardeners use to grow seedlings, with fine holes in the bottom for drainage). When germinating very tiny seeds such as alfalfa you will need to line your seed tray with damp, plain white kitchen towels. Place the trays inside a larger tray to catch the water that drains from them. Soak the seeds/ grains/pulses overnight, as in the jar method, then rinse them well and spread them a few layers deep in each of the trays. Spray the seeds with water (by putting them under the tap or by using a spray bottle) and leave in a warm place. Check the seeds each day and spray them again if they seem dry. If the seeds get too wet they will rot, so be careful not to overwater them. Larger seeds such as chickpeas, lentils and mung beans need to be gently turned over with your hand once a day to ensure that the seeds underneath are not suffocated. Alfalfa seeds can be simply sprinkled on damp paper towels and left alone and after four or five days will have grown into a thick green carpet. Don't forget to put alfalfa sprouts in some sunlight for a day or so to develop lots of chlorophyll. When the seeds are ready, harvest them, rinse them well in a sieve and put them in an airtight container or sealed polythene bag until you want them. To make the next batch, rinse the trays well and begin again.

Tips and tricks

Some sprouts are more difficult to grow than others, but usually if seeds fail to germinate it is because they are too old and no longer viable. It is always worth buying top-quality seeds because, after removing dead and broken seeds, and taking germinating failures into account, they work out better value than cheaper ones. Also try to avoid seeds treated with insecticide/ fungicide mixtures such as those which are sold in gardening shops and some nurseries. Healthfood shops and wholefood emporia are usually your best bet. At the latter you can buy seeds very cheaply for sprouting in bulk. It is fun to experiment with growing all kinds of sprouts from radish seeds to soya beans, but avoid plants whose greens are known to be poisonous such as the deadly nightshade family, potato and tomato seeds. Also avoid kidney beans, as they are poisonous raw.

Some of the easiest to begin with are alfalfa seeds, adzuki (aduki) beans, mung beans, lentils, fenugreek seeds, radish seeds, chickpeas and wheat. Others include sunflower seeds, pumpkin seeds, sesame seeds, buckwheat, flax, mint, red clover and triticale. These latter can sometimes be difficult to find or to sprout – the 'seeds' must be in their hulls and the nuts must be really fresh and undamaged. Good luck!

Variety	Soak Time Measure	Dry Harvest	Days to Tips	Sprouting
Alfalfa	Overnight	3 tbsp	4–5	Grow on wet paper towel – place in light for last 24 hrs
Chickpea	Up to 24 hours	2 cups	3–4	Needs long soak, renew water twice during soak
Fenugreek	Overnight	1/2 cup	3–5	Pungent flavour
Lentil	Overnight	1 cup	3–5	Earthy flavour
Mung	Overnight	3/4 cup	3–5	Grow in the dark – place in light for last 24 hours

Sprouting Cereal Grasses

You will need:
   A seed-tray (a kitchen tray will do)
   Good organic potting compost
   8–10 layers of newspaper
   A sheet of plastic to cover the tray
   Seed – hard red winter wheat or buckwheat, barley etc.

How to sprout:

1. Soak approximately 1 cup of seed for 12 hours in water (cover well), pour off the water and allow to drain for 12 hours.
2. Half-fill the seed-tray with compost (so that the compost comes half-way up the sides of the tray), level the surface and spray with a fine spray. Make sure you do not soak the compost.
3. Place the soaked seeds on the wet soil so that the seeds are evenly spread and not on top of each other.
4. Soak the newspaper thoroughly, cut to the size of the seed tray and cover the seeds. Place the plastic on top of the newspaper.
5. Leave the tray in a well-ventilated, not over-warm room for 3 days.
6. At the end of 3 days remove the plastic and newspaper and put the trays somewhere where they will get plenty of light – a sunny windowsill, for instance – and water once a day, making sure you do not soak the soil.
7. In about 5–8 days the plants should be 15–20cm (6–8"), high standing upright and nicely green. They are then ready to cut.
8. Cut the greens close to the soil with a sharp knife. They can be kept in the fridge in plastic bags for several days.

Cereal grasses can be grown all the year round wherever you live and regardless of whether you have a garden. Use organic seed, which should be available from good healthfood stores. Cereal grasses can only be juiced using a machine specifically designed for this purpose.

Alternatively they can be put into a powerful blender such as the Vita-Mix with ½ cup of raw fresh juice or spring water and blended for 10–20 seconds to pulverize them. Then you need to strain away the indigestible cellulose before serving.

Further Reading

Good Diet

The Bircher-Benner Health Guide, Ruth Kunz-Bircher, Unwin Paperbacks, London, 1981.

Nutrition for Vegetarians, Agatha Moody Thrash M.D. & Calvin L. Thrash M.D., Thrash Publications, Seale, Alabama, 1982.

Nutrition and Physical Degeneration, Weston A. Price, Price-Pottenger Nutritional Foundation, La Mesa, California, 1970.

The Prevention of Incurable Disease, M. Bircher-Benner, James Clarke & Co, Cambridge, 1981.

Nutrition Against Disease, R. Williams, Pitman Publishing Co., New York, 1971.

Life in the Twentieth Century, Richard Taska Jr., Omangod Press, Woodstock Valley, Connecticut, 1981.

Eating Your Way to Health, Ruth Bircher-Benner, Faber and Faber, London, 1961.

Dr Bircher-Benner's Way to Positive Health and Vitality 1867–1967, Verlag Bircher-Benner Erlenback, Zürich, Switzerland, 1967.

Diet and Salad Suggestions, N.W. Walker, Norwalk Press, Arizona, 1940.

Macrobiotic Diet, Michio & Aveline Kushi, Japan Publications, Tokyo and New York, 1993.

Subtle Energies in Foods

The Electromagnetic Energy in Foods, Dr Hazel Parcells, Par-X-Cell School of Scientific Nutrition, Albuquerque, New Mexico, 1974.

Man and Biologically Active Substances, I. I. Brekhman, Pergamon Press, Oxford, 1980.

The Phenomena of Life: A Radio-Electrical Interpretation, George Crile, W. W. Norton, New York, 1936.

A Cancer Therapy, Max Gerson, Totality Books, Del Mar, California, 1977.

What Is Life? and *Mind and Matter?*, Erwin Schrödinger, Cambridge University Press, 1980.

Food Science for All, M.O. Bircher-Benner, C.W. Daniel, London, 1928.

The Essene Science of Life, E.B. Szekely, International Biogenic Society, Cartago, Costa Rica, 1978.

Green Foods and Drinks

The Magic of Green Buckwheat, Kate Spencer, Romany Herb Products Limited, 1987.

Real Health Starts with Eating Light, Mitsuo Koda M.D., privately published.

The Wheatgrass Book, Ann Wigmore, Avery Publishing Group Inc, Wayne, New Jersey, 1985.

Cereal Grass, Ed., Ronald L. Seibold, M.S., Keats Publishing Inc, New Canaan, Connecticut, 1991.

Wheatgrass Juice, Betsey Russell Manning, Greensward Press, Calistoga, California, 1994.

Chlorella, Dr David Steenblock, Aging Research Institute, El Toro, California, 1987.

Why George Should Eat Broccoli, Paul A. Stitt, The Dougherty Company, Milwaukee, Wisconsin, 1990.

Nature's Healing Grasses, H.E. Kirchner, H.C. White Publications, Riverside, California, date unknown.

Wild Foods
Wild Food, Roger Phillips, Orbis Publishing, London, 1983.

Rejuvenation
Become Younger, N.W. Walker, D.Sc., Norwalk Press, Phoenix, Arizona, 1949.

The New Ageless Ageing, Leslie Kenton, Vermilion, London, 1995.

Therapeutic Use of Juice and Foods
Encyclopaedia of Healing Juices, John Heinerman, Parker Publishing Company, New York, 1994.

Total Juicing, Elaine LaLanne with Richard Beyno, Plume, Penguin Books, USA, 1992.

Food Power, George Schwartz, M.D., McGraw-Hill Book Company, New York, 1979.

Food Enzymes & Health
Enzymes & Enzyme Therapy, Anthony J. Cichoke, D.C., Keats Publishing Inc., New Canaan, Connecticut, 1994.

Enzyme Nutrition, Dr Edward Howell, Avery Publishing Group Inc., Wayne, New Jersey, 1985.

Enzymes The Foundation of Life, D.A Lopez, M.D., R.M. Williams, M.D., Ph.D., M. Miehlke, M.D., The Neville Press Inc., Charleston, S.C., 1994.

'A Turning Point in Nutritional Science', R. Bircher, reprint from *Lee Foundation for Nutritional Research*, No. 80, Milwaukee, Wisconsin.

The New Raw Energy, Leslie & Susannah Kenton, Vermilion, London, 1994.

Juices & Juicing
Raw Vegetable Juices, N.W. Walker, Jove/Harcourt Brace Jovanovich, New York, 1977.

Index

acidity 29, 187, 248, 268
   acid fruit 96, 237
acne 247, 269
additives 53, 57, 182, 248
adrenal glands 252
adzuki beans: sprouting
   82, 385, 422
ageing 180, 221–2
AHA fruit acids 237
alfalfa 261; dish-salad 356;
   Father of All Juices 289;
   sprouting 80, 81, 82, 86,
   384, 22, 436
alcohol 261, 323, 328–34
alkalinity 29, 96–7, 248
allergies and sensitivities
   29, 30, 43, 83, 247–8,
   250–2, 255, 258, 345–6,
   352, 389, 428
almonds: Almond Apple
   Porridge 105–6;
   Fermented Seed Loaf
   408; Italian Pesto 381;
   Mange-tout and Almond
   Stir-fry 150; Nut-Milk
   Shake 351; Sweet Treats
   394–5
aluminium 388; utensils
   343–4
amino acids 47–8, 71, 367,
   382
anaemia 248–9
anise seeds 382
antibiotics 82
anti-oxidants 8, 181, 192,
   221, 222, 258–9
appetite 45, 50, 63, 70
apple juice 189, 194–5,
   342, 401, 403; Apple
   Zinger 290; with carrot
   194–5, 292; with celery
   and fennel 290; Easy
   Does It 295; Fatty Acid
   Frolic 295–6; Green
   Friend 297; Green Wild
   298; Green Wow 298;
   Les lie's Cocktail 300;
   Linusit Perfect 300–1;
   with pears 289–90; with
   pears and berries 290;
   spicy 309

apple mint 377–8
apple seeds 197
apples 65, 388; Almond
   Apple Porridge 105–6;
   apple and cinnamon tea
   402; Apple Ginger Salad
   370–1; Apple Raspberry
   Frappé 108–9; Carob
   and Apple Cake 395;
   Live Apple Sauce 105;
   Snappy Apple Salad 103;
   see also apple juice
apricots, dried 424; Apricot
   Lhassi 107; Apricot
   Shake 351; Spiked
   Apricot Supreme 101;
   Winter Muesli 348
arrame 68
arthritis 249–51, 394, 430
artichokes 152–3, 372
Asparagus Soup Raw 144
asthma 251–2
Atomic Lift-Off 290–1
Aubergine Paté 156–7
avidin 428
avocados: Avocado Citrus
   Salad 370; Avocado
   Delight 135; Avocado
   Smoothie 320; Avocado-
   Tomato Dresing 318;
   Bio-active Avocado and
   Tomato Soup 142;
   Curried Avocado Dip-
   dressing 357; Fresh
   Green Soup 406–7;
   stuffed 104

bacteria, yoghurt 82, 87
Baked Vegetables 159
bananas 95, 98, 256, 257;
   Banana-Coconut-Mint
   Frappé 109; Banana and
   Honeydew with Apricot
   326; Banana Muesli 348;
   Banana Shake 398;
   Creamy Date Delight
   109; dried 424; juicing
   324; Leslie's Cocktail
   300; Raspberry and
   Banana Pie Filling 409;
   Rocky Road Bananas

396; Smoothies 324,
   325; Yoghurt Shake 351
barley 421; Barley
   Mushroom Soup 140–1;
   Barley Pilaff 165–6;
   Barley Roasts 372;
   cooking 414; Scottish
   Barley Soup 144–5;
   sprouting 386
basil 376
bean curd, see tofu
beans see pulses
beetroot 189, 198; Beet
   Treat 210–11, 291; Beetroot, Carrot and Orange
   291; Borscht 416–17;
   Devil's Delight 121;
   Dracula's Delight 358;
   Flamingo Soup 321; Red
   Cool 306; Red Devil 306;
   Red Genius 307; as
   salad sprinkle 372
Bellini 329
berries 195–6, 249; Berry
   Muesli 106
beta-carotene 192, 223,
   224, 258–9
binge eating 44
Bioactive Avocado and
   Tomato Soup 142
bioflavonoids 37, 196,
   252, 258
biophoton radiation 35
biotin 428
Bircher-Benner, Max 8, 33,
   34, 35, 175, 225, 346–7
biscuits 70; Shortcake 395
blackberries: Blackberry
   Sorbet 397; Pineapple
   and Blackberry Frappé
   108
blenders, food 61, 62, 342
bloating 83, 97, 215, 234
blood-sugar levels 188,
   242, 262, 263–4, 388
Bloody Mary, Ultimate 334
Blue Dolphin Salad 114
Blueberry Muffins 240
body building 218–29
boredom 206, 216
boron 68